DALTON
HARDCASTLE

DISORDERS
OF
FLUENCY

STUDIES IN DISORDERS OF COMMUNICATION

SECOND EDITION

W

WHURR PUBLISHER

LONDON   JERSEY CITY

© Whurr Publishers Limited 1989

First published 1977 by
Edward Arnold (Publishers) Ltd
Second edition 1989 published by
Cole and Whurr Limited
Reprinted 1990 (twice) by Whurr Publishers Limited
19b Compton Terrace, London N1 2UN

British Library Cataloguing in Publication Data

Dalton, Peggy
  Disorders of fluency and their effects on communication.—2nd
  ed.
  1. Fluency disorders.
  I. Title   II. Hardcastle, W.J.   III. Series
  616.85′5

ISBN: 1 871381 07 X

Printed and bound in Great Britain by Athenaeum Press Ltd, Newcastle upon Tyne

Contents

General preface

This series is the first to approach the problem of language disability as a single field. It attempts to bring together areas of study which have traditionally been treated under separate headings, and to focus on the common problems of analysis, assessment and treatment which characterize them. Its scope therefore includes the specifically linguistic aspects of the work of such areas as speech therapy, remedial teaching, teaching of the deaf and educational psychology, as well as those aspects of mother-tongue and foreign-language teaching which pose similar problems. The research findings and practical techniques from each of these fields can inform the others, and we hope one of the main functions of this series will be to put people from one profession into contact with the analogous situations found in others.

It is therefore not a series about specific syndromes or educationally narrow problems. While the orientation of a volume is naturally towards a single main area, and reflects an author's background, it is editorial policy to ask authors to consider the implications of what they say for the fields with which they have not been primarily concerned. Nor is this a series about disability in general. The medical, social, educational and other factors which enter into a comprehensive evaluation of any problems will not be studied as ends in themselves, but only in so far as they bear directly on the understanding of the nature of the language behaviour involved. The aim is to provide a much needed emphasis on the description and analysis of language as such, and on the provision of specific techniques of therapy or remediation. In this way, we hope to bridge the gap between the theoretical discussion of 'causes' and the practical tasks of treatment—two sides of language disability which it is uncommon to see systematically related.

Despite restricting the area of disability to specifically linguistic matters—and in particular emphasizing problems of the production and comprehension of spoken language—it should be clear that the series' scope goes considerably beyond this. For the first books, we have selected topics which have been particularly neglected in recent years, and which seem most able to benefit from contemporary research in linguistics and its related disciplines, English studies, psychology, sociology and education. Each volume will put its subject matter in perspective, and will provide an introductory slant to its presentation. In this way, we hope to provide specialized studies which can be used as texts for components of teaching courses, as well as material that is directly applicable to the needs of professional workers. It is also hoped that this orientation will place the series within the reach of the interested layman—in particular, the parents or family of the linguistically disabled.

David Crystal
Jean Cooper

Preface

Any discussion of disfluency and the effects it may have on communication is hampered by the absence of a clearly defined concept of fluency in speech. It is accepted that 'normal' nonfluency exists in the utterance of all speakers, varying with the context, the emotional state of the speaker and the complexity of what is being said. Yet the point at which disruption can be considered pathological is, for the most part, determined in a highly subjective way. In more severe cases of stuttering, cluttering, dysarthric and dyspraxic speech disfluency is readily recognized by both speaker and listener as disturbing the expression of ideas and the perception of what is being said. In milder cases, however, it may only be the speaker who is aware of difficulty. He may, in fact, be far more fluent than another whose utterance is continually broken by pauses and repetitions, which may distract his audience but of which he is unaware.

We have begun this book, therefore, with an introductory section on the general problem of fluency itself. This is followed in chapter 2 by an outline of the stages involved in speech production. Five basic functions are discussed: ideation, neurolinguistic program-planning, the motor regulator function and monitoring. In chapter 3 some factors involved in the evaluation of fluency are considered in the light of research findings from a wide range of disciplines. Speech variables, such as transition smoothness, pausing, rhythmical patterning and overall tempo are examined in detail and some of their manifestations described as they affect fluency in both normal and pathological speech.

The second part of the book is mainly concerned with those disorders considered to be specific fluency problems, namely stuttering and cluttering. But some consideration is also given to the effects on communication of the neurologically based disabilities, dysarthria and articulatory dyspraxia. Although the term 'stammering' is more familiar to many British readers, we have chosen 'stuttering' for use in this volume, since it is more widely accepted internationally. In chapter 4 an outline is given of the main theories as to the nature and cause of stuttering. We have added to our discussion of views on the subject found in the literature, those commonly held by the stutterers themselves and those with whom they communicate.

In chapter 5 an attempt has been made to trace the development of disfluency in children. The growth of stuttering behaviours is studied and the effects of disfluency on attitudes towards communication. Chapter 6 extends the discussion of

the overt manifestations of stuttering and its psychological aspects into the context of adult life. Problems involved in the assessment of stuttering are considered
and suggestions made as to the basic requirements of an evaluation of this type
of disfluency. Evidence of the effects of stuttering on communication is drawn both
from experimental work and information provided by the speakers themselves.
Current treatment approaches are then outlined.

In our section on cluttering in chapter 7 traditional views, particularly of the
personality of the clutterer, are questioned and the relationship between cluttering
and stuttering reconsidered in the light of more recent work. The links between
cluttering and disfluency associated with neurological disease, especially Parkinson's, are discussed. Dysarthria and articulatory dyspraxia are briefly considered
for their effects on speech fluency, although more usually viewed as disorders of
articulation, and the effects on communication of these disabilities are tentatively
suggested in the absence of experimental data.

Throughout this book we have attempted to relate disorders of fluency to
ideas from many disciplines concerning fluency and normal nonfluency and to assess
the effects of disfluency on communication as a whole. In the course of this study,
areas have been highlighted where our knowledge is scanty and remediation
procedures based on too little experimental data. Our final chapter outlines some
suggestions for future work which could lead to a greater understanding of the
problems involved in these disorders. We stress not only the need for more research,
but the need for findings to be related more fully and for those who work directly
with these disabilities to exchange ideas to a far greater extent than at present.

We should like to thank David Crystal and Jean Cooper for their helpful
criticisms as editors of this series and Peter Roach, Paul Fletcher, Margaret Fawcus
and Rosemarie Helps for their comments on some of the chapters. To many of the
people who have come to the City Literary Institute we are especially grateful, not
only for all we have learned about stuttering from working with them but for the
insights they have given us into the problem from the stutterer's point of view.

September 1976   PD
                                                                 WJH

Preface to second edition

Our first edition consisted of two fairly distinct parts, with chapters 1–3 giving the background in terms of a discussion of the nature of fluency, a model of speech production and some variables involved in an evaluation of fluency. The rest of the book was concerned with the disorders themselves and their effects on communication for both speaker and listener

In this second edition we have updated the background section by including a new chapter 4. In this chapter we have brought together recent work on the quantitative measurement of stuttering in the clinic and have incorporated some of these measures in a new profiling procedure which aims to identify the main phonetic, phonological, prosodic and linguistic characteristics of a given speaker's disfluency. The speech of a severe stutterer is profiled, using this new procedure and the clinical implications both for treatment and for evaluating progress are discussed.

Part Two has also been extended by the inclusion of a new chapter — 10 — on developments in the understanding of stuttering and cluttering. In preparing this chapter we were mindful of the fact that much of the focus of research and the literature in the last decade has been on broader issues of assessment and therapy and there has been growing concern over the problem of maintenance of the behavioural and psychological changes brought about through treatment. Our major emphases in Part Two, therefore, lie on advances in the comprehensive assessment of the persons involved, the contexts in which they live and factors affecting the outcome of therapy.

1

The problem of fluency

The concept of fluency

In popular usage, the terms 'fluent' and 'fluency' normally refer to a general proficiency in the act of speaking or writing. According to the Oxford English Dictionary, for example, fluency means 'a smooth and easy flow; readiness, smoothness esp. with regard to speech'; and 'readiness of utterance, flow of words'. A fluent speaker is said to be one who is 'ready in the use of words, able to express himself readily and easily in speech or writing'. Odhams Dictionary of the English Language (Smith and O'Loughlin 1946) offers a similar definition of fluent: 'having a ready command and flow of words; voluble, glib; spoken easily, rapidly, and without hesitation; flowing, smoothly and continuous; proceeding readily and naturally without effort.' In these definitions the temporal and sequential features of speech are emphasized; these may cover a considerably wide range including 'breaks' in the 'smooth flow of speech' such as pauses, interruptions etc., and repetitions of linguistic elements such as sounds, syllables, words and phrases. In addition, factors such as rhythmical patterning, stress and intonation characteristics and overall rate of utterance could be considered relevant features in an assessment of fluency.

The term 'fluency' is used slightly differently in the context of language learning. Here fluency is used to describe a level of efficiency in a foreign language. A person popularly described as a fluent speaker of French, for example, 'is one who possesses the ability to express himself like a native speaker of French', to 'think in the foreign language' or to 'have a good command of the language'. (See further Leeson 1975). The latter quality, that of having a good command of the language, perhaps implies somewhat more than efficiency in speech and writing only; it may imply in addition an ability in comprehending the language (Crystal 1971). However, in the normal use of the term fluency in language teaching, emphasis is placed on the production side of speech communication.

There seems to be more involved in an assessment of fluency in a foreign language than the temporal and sequential aspects of the speech process. Accuracy in the use of the language is another potentially important factor to consider and will include such features as correct adherence to the phonological, syntactic and semantic rules of the language, to prosodic variables such as stress and intonation patterns, as well as to the use of appropriate vocabulary. Thus the main factors contributing to fluency in the foreign-language-learning context can be grouped under two main headings: those relating to accuracy in the use of the language, and (somewhat more specifically) those relating to temporal and sequential aspects of the speech output, such as repetitions and pauses. Various attempts to measure fluency in foreign language speaking (e.g. Husén 1969) have taken account of these two main aspects using scores such as 'number of propositions (clauses) in the responses; number of propositions with correct structures; number of propositions exhibiting one or more hesitations; number of propositions with correct vocabulary' etc. There is clearly a real difficulty in establishing guidelines for 'correctness' in this context. For example, correctness will depend crucially on the particular stylistic context of the utterance. What may be a perfectly acceptable linguistic form in one style may be quite inappropriate in another. An obvious example would be in the use of vocabulary. Colloquial forms such as slang and swear words, although regarded as normal in spontaneous conversational speech with one's peers, would usually be quite unsuitable in the context of a formal lecture situation. And even in a particular stylistic context there are problems in deciding and evaluating the limits of acceptability (cf. Quirk and Svartvik 1966).

Another criterion which has been used in an evaluation of fluency in language teaching is the 'quantity' or 'amount' of language material spoken or written within a given time. This criterion was used in the scoring procedure mentioned above where the indices 'number of clauses in the responses' and 'number of different grammatical structures represented in the response' (for 30 sec.) were used for speaking fluency, and 'the completeness (or amount written)' for writing fluency. Once again stylistic variations will be crucially important, at least as far as speaking fluency tests are concerned—there being presumably a fairly close relationship between the style and overall utterance tempo.

In the field of speech therapy, the term fluency is normally used in the context of disorders of fluency, specifically those disorders commonly called stuttering and cluttering. Both these disorders are manifested primarily by impairments in the temporal and sequential aspects of speech output. Stuttering manifestations may include, for example, repetitions (of sounds, syllables, words and phrases), and 'blocks' or 'hard contacts' (Van Riper 1954) which involve obstruction to the airflow caused by abnormally high tension in the articulatory or laryngeal muscles. Phonetically, a hard contact may be described as a tensely articulated closure phase of a stop consonant, or as a glottal stop initiation of vowel sounds. Both the repetitions and blocks may affect the normal rhythmical patterning of speech. Cluttering may have some of the manifestations of stuttering but is characterized specifically by 'uncontrolled speed of utterance resulting in truncated, dysrhythmic and incoherent utterance' (College of Speech Therapists 1959). We shall be discussing these disorders in more detail in the latter part of this volume, where attention will be focused not only on the overt phonetic and linguistic manifestations of these disorders by the speaker, but on the whole complex of psychological factors which operate in both the speaker and listener potentially to affect the communication situation. We shall discuss also how disfluency features may affect communication in patients with other types of speech and language disorders, such as some of the dysarthrias, with neuromuscular impairment of the speech system, and aphasia, with a disturbance of central language processing.

The assessment of fluency

What factors are involved in an assessment of fluency? Obviously it is important to know in what ways fluency can potentially be disturbed before we can begin to evaluate a speech disorder as being primarily a disorder of fluency. In a discussion of fluency in stutterers and non-stutterers by Johnson (1961) a number of factors were suggested as potentially important for evaluation. These included, in a given speech utterance, the number of interjections of sounds, syllables, words or phrases; the number of repetitions of words, parts of words and phrases; the number of revisions, incomplete phrases and broken words; and the number of prolonged sounds. For a more complete picture of the temporal and sequential features potentially affecting an evaluation of fluency, one could add to this list features related to the location, distribution and frequency of pauses, to the rhythmical patterning (e.g. regularity of the occurrence of stressed beats in a passage (see chapter 3)), to intonation and stress characteristics, and to overall rate of utterance. In a discussion of ways in which fluency may be measured, Minifie and Cooker (1964) suggest there are two basic types of disfluencies: 'disfluencies of syllable insertion' including repetitions, revisions and interjections, and 'disfluencies of deliberation' including pauses and prolongations. The authors state that 'disfluencies of deliberation interrupt patterns of fluency by adding to the total amount of time required to read a given passage. Disfluencies of syllable insertion not only consume time, but also add to the total number of sounds uttered while reading a given passage' (p. 190). The authors propose a 'disfluency index' expressed by the ratio $\dfrac{S}{W/M}$ where S equals the total number of syllables uttered in a passage and W/M equals the rate of utterance calculated in words per minute. In applying the index to a comparison of a group of stutterers and a group of normal speakers they found that although some stutterers received disfluency scores within the range obtained by normal speakers, stutterers in general received much larger disfluency scores. One of the major difficulties in evaluating speech as pathologically disfluent lies in the fact that many of the features characteristic of a disfluency problem also apply to normal speech. Normal speech, in fact, particularly spontaneous conversational speech, is far from fluent in the sense of 'smoothly flowing', without hesitations etc. Goldman-Eisler (1968, 31) points out that spontaneous speech is 'a highly fragmented and discontinuous activity. When even at its most fluent, two-thirds of spoken language comes in chunks of less than six words, the attributes of flow and fluency in spontaneous speech must be judged an illusion.' Goldman-Eisler was referring primarily to gaps or discontinuities occurring in the speech signal resulting from hesitation pauses. But there are many other features other than pauses contributing to 'normal nonfluency'. These include for example interruptions, anacolutha, loosely coordinated clauses (see Crystal and Davy 1969, Crystal 1971) as well as temporal and sequential 'aberrations' such as hesitations (either filled with an intrusive sound such as 'er' [ə:] or 'um' [ʌm] or unfilled (i.e. silent)), repetitions, elisions etc. Many of these features were used in the disfluency measurements of investigators such as Johnson (1961),

Johnson, Darley and Spriesterbach (1963) and others. It is not surprising, then, that in their comparisons of the speech of stutterers and normals, considerable overlap was found for some of the disfluency categories, for example, broken words and repetition of words. It is also interesting to note that in an investigation by Boehmler (1958) into listener responses to nonfluencies, features such as repetitions of sounds or syllables were classified by listeners as pathological stuttering more often than were other kinds of disfluencies. These were features not noted by Johnson (1961) as overlapping with the normative data. An investigation by Yairi and Clifton (1972) discusses the typical breakdowns of fluency in three groups of normal speakers: preschool children, high-school seniors and geriatric persons. They list seven 'disfluency types': interjections, part-word repetitions, word repetitions, phrase repetitions, revision-incomplete phrases, dysrhythmic phonation and tense pauses. An analysis of the distribution of disfluency types per 100 words for each of the subject groups showed that in general there is a decrease in total disfluency from preschool to high-school age, and an increase in disfluency from high school to the geriatric group. Disfluency types most prevalent in all groups were interjections, word repetitions and revision-incomplete phrases.

In his discussion of the overlap in disfluency features for his stuttering and normal subjects, Johnson (1961) points to the need to consider the communication situation as a whole where not only speech and language features of the speaker are to be considered but also reactions from the listener. As he puts it:

> The varying degrees of overlapping of the distributions of disfluency measures for the subjects classified as stutterers and those not so classified imply that the problem called stuttering is not to be adequately identified or defined solely by reference to speech disfluency as such. It is suggested that variables associated with the perceptual and evaluative reactions of the listener and of the speaker, as well as those associated with the frequencies and forms of disfluency of the speaker are to be included in an adequately comprehensive and systematic consideration of the problem called stuttering. (20)

We shall be emphasizing throughout this volume the need to consider fluency features as they affect communication as a whole, i.e. as affecting both speaker and listener.

Despite attempts to quantify fluency in terms of speech variables such as those mentioned above, the concept of fluency remains rather vague and ill-defined. This is partly because of the wide variety of phonetic and linguistic features potentially contributing to an evaluation of fluency, and also partly because as yet no suitable experimental evidence is available as to how one might assess the relative importance of the various categories of fluency. As Crystal (1971, 51) points out, far more is involved than simply temporal aspects such as hesitancy. He mentions the following as potential factors influencing an evaluation of fluency: syntactic features such as inter-sentence connecting devices (e.g. introductory adverbials), prosodic features of speech such as the use of hesitation and tempo, pitch range, loudness and rhythmicality variation as well as intonation patterns.

One way of shedding light on the problem is to examine closely the main speech features involved in an assessment of fluency, and the various ways these features can be affected in normal speech. Most of these features can be subsumed under a general concept of *transition smoothness*, which may operate at a number of different levels: at the (segmental) phonetic level between speech sounds and syllables; at the grammatical level between phrases, clauses, sentences etc.; at the prosodic level between intonation units such as tone groups; and at the lexical/ semantic level between thematic elements or 'sense groups' in a discourse. In discussing the various manifestations of transition smoothness, we have found the following variables to be particularly useful:

pausing (i.e. discontinuities of gaps in the speech audio signal due for example to articulatory closures, hesitation and juncture pauses)
rhythmical patterning (the regular succession of stressed 'beats' in a speech utterance)
regulation of tempo
intonation and stress patterns
other features including interjections, interruptions etc., which cannot be easily included under the other categories.

A breakdown in fluency, whether a pathological disfluency or a normal nonfluency, can be regarded primarily as a breakdown in transition smoothness (the phonetic manifestations of stuttering, for example, have been described in this way by some investigators (e.g. Wingate 1969b)) and may be manifested by a variety of different features: at the phonetic level by repetitions (e.g. of sounds and syllables), or by prolongations of sound segments; at the grammatical level by loss of coordinating conjunctions etc.; at the prosodic level by, for example, a succession of similar stereotyped intonation patterns; and at the lexical/semantic level by the break-down in the logical sequence of ideas in a discourse. As far as pausing is concerned, disfluency may be manifested by too many and abnormally long pauses or by pauses at inappropriate places. Rhythmical patterning, regulation in overall rate of utterance, and stress and intonation characteristics, also, may be potentially affected in disfluent speech. A lack of intonational variations in an utterance ('monotony'), for example, may be considered a potential feature contributing to disfluency (Crystal 1971).

The general concept of transition smoothness and the main characteristics of variations in pausing, rhythmical patterning and regulation of utterance rate will be discussed in more detail in chapter 3. We shall describe, for example, some of the factors which may affect these features in normal speech and so provide a framework in which to discuss those pathological disfluencies characteristic of such disorders as stuttering and cluttering. In chapter 2, also, we shall be concerned primarily with the normal rather than the pathological situation in discussing some of the neural functions involved in the generation of a speech utterance. We shall see in the latter part of the volume how some of these neural functions may be affected in the various disorders of fluency. As we mentioned earlier in this chapter, one of our primary concerns throughout this work will be the differences between pathological disfluencies and features of normal nonfluency. In many cases we will find this difference is mainly one of degree rather than of kind. For example, stutterers frequently pause longer between clauses than do normal speakers, and most aphasics pause longer and more frequently (Quinting 1971). In some cases, however, the disfluent manifestation will be of a type uncharacteristic of normal speech. For example, a prolongation of sounds caused by a 'hard block' accompanied by increased muscular tension in the articulatory and laryngeal muscles is a characteristic of many stutterers but would be extremely unusual in normal speech. This latter manifestation, that of the hard block, also affects communication as a whole, because the listener is normally immediately aware of the considerable discomfort the stutterer is experiencing at the moment of blocking. The psychological pressures exerted on the pathologically disfluent speaker in the normal communication situation will be explored more fully in chapters 7 and 8.

This volume consists basically of two main parts. In the first part (chapters 1 to 4), we shall be bringing together some of the research findings from a relatively wide variety of disciplines including speech therapy, phonetics, linguistics, language teaching, psychology and sociology to provide an outline of the main factors contributing to an evaluation of fluency. In the second part of the volume (chapters 5 to 9) those disorders usually considered to be specific disfluency problems, namely stuttering and cluttering, are discussed. In these latter chapters we discuss various theories of stuttering and cluttering, the developmental aspects of stuttering in children and the overt phonetic and linguistic manifestations of the disorder in adults. Throughout the book we shall stress that in these and many other speech and language disorders (such as the dysarthrias, dyspraxia and some forms of aphasia), disruption of fluency is a feature affecting communication as a whole, both for speaker and listener.

2

Some aspects of a preliminary model of speech production

In chapter 1 we discussed some of the different ways of looking at fluency and saw how pathological disfluency was characterized mainly by some impairment in the temporal organization of speech production. In order to place our discussion of speech fluency in some sort of theoretical framework, it is important to outline some of the main functions the brain performs in the production of a normal speech utterance. This framework will then serve as a theoretical basis for the discussion of the pathological situation which follows in later chapters. Most of the discussion in this chapter will be rather speculative in view of the inaccessibility of the human brain to direct experimental investigation; however, a great deal of important information about central neural processes can be inferred from studying details of the speech output, such as the dynamics of articulatory activity. The research strategy of inferring central unobservable processes by examining the output is by no means without precedent and is regarded as an acceptable research procedure (Beveridge 1961). As Laver (1970, 61) points out, 'If we want to know how the brain controls speech, we must first look at speech itself.' The model of speech production discussed in this chapter is based closely on that proposed by Laver in a series of articles (1968, 1969, 1970, 1977).

For the purposes of exposition it is convenient to discuss five basic functions or stages involved in the generation of a speech utterance:

an *ideation* function, where a central underlying idea or intention to say something is first initiated;

a *neurolinguistic program*[1] *planning function*, where the expression of the idea takes shape in terms of the phonological, syntactic and semantic rules of the language, and where words are selected from a lexical storage system;

a *motor regulator* function, where the neurolinguistic program is converted into temporal sequences of motor commands to the appropriate speech muscles;

a *myodynamic execution* function, where the articulatory, laryngeal and respiratory organs carry out the sequence of movements designated by the motor regulator;

a *monitoring* function, where 'errors' at various stages in the speech generation process, whether at the program-planning level or at the myodynamic execution level, are detected, and appropriate strategies adopted for their correction.

[1] The word 'program' is a term borrowed from computer science and is normally used in this context with the American spelling.

Broadly speaking, there is some sort of logical temporal progression in these different functions, with the ideation function and the program-planning function preceding the motor regulator and myodynamic execution functions. The monitoring system is rather more difficult to fit into this temporal progression, as it can presumably operate at all levels continuously. That is, monitoring systems may be important both at the myodynamic execution level in checking whether the articulatory activity is appropriate for a given plan (here the feedback of sensory information from receptor organs in the oral mucosa, muscles and joints plays an important role), and also at a 'higher', more abstract level, checking the appropriateness of the neurolinguistic program for expression of the original idea or intention. And as we shall see later in this chapter, monitoring may be proceeding *continuously* at the 'lower' motor levels involving feedback of sensory information.

There is presumably also some progression fiom the ideation to the myodynamic execution stage in the degree of voluntariness on the part of the speaker. The ideation and program-planning functions are concerned with potentially complex cognitive activities and probably involve the cerebral cortex of the brain, while the motor regulator and execution functions are concerned with largely automatic specification of motor commands and movements of speech organs following the pattern of motor activity prescribed at the program-planning stages. The monitoring function presumably occurs at all levels of the brain and utilizes neural structures such as the cerebellum, thalamus and cerebral cortex. Automatic monitoring of the speech activity occurs outside the speaker's voluntary control and probably involves primarily 'lower' structures such as the cerebellum; whereas conscious monitoring presumably involves 'higher' neural structures such as the cerebral cortex.

The main characteristics of these five main functions will be discussed now in some detail.

Ideation function

During the ideation stage of the speech-encoding process, an abstract underlying idea or intention of the speaker to say something is first initiated. Because of the potentially great complexity of cognitive activity involved in the ideation stage it probably takes place in the pre-frontal zones of the cerebral cortex of the speaker (see Luria 1973), and will be contingent upon a wide variety of factors such as the speaker's past experience and details of the prevailing situation. The degree of cognitive complexity involved in the ideation stage will vary enormously; Hughlings Jackson (1932) was one of the first to differentiate 'propositional' speech, such as the expression of abstract concepts involving some degree of complexity, from more 'automatic' speech such as greetings, clichés etc.

The speaker's task is to formulate an appropriate neurolinguistic plan or strategy for the expression of the original idea or intention, although just how we go about this process is at present unknown. We can assume however that, during the language acquisition stage, a child may be faced with a relatively large number of alternate plans for a given initial idea and that after some practice in the formulation and execution of different strategies, a particular optimal plan soon becomes preferred to all others (cf. Bernstein 1967). In order that we can test the suitability of a plan for expression of the initial idea it is presumably necessary for the idea to be retained for a short period of time while a feedback monitoring process assesses the plan's acceptability (see below).

Neurolinguistic program-planning function

The neurolinguistic program for the idea initiated at the ideation stage can be regarded as a sort of blueprint of the phonological, syntactic and semantic characteristics of the speech utterance. It is likely that the program-planning function is hierarchically organized, with smaller structures such as words and syllables operating within larger structures such as clauses, sentences and paragraphs. Lashley (1951) sees this hierarchical organization as characteristic of all voluntary behaviour and states:

> I have devoted so much time to discussion of the problem of syntax not only because language is one of the most important products of human cerebral action, but also because the problems raised by the organization of language seem to me to be characteristic of almost all other cerebral activity. There is a series of hierarchies of organization, the order of vocal movements in pronouncing the words, the order of words in the sentence, the order of sentences in the paragraph, the rational order of paragraphs in a discourse. Not only speech, but all skilled acts seem to involve the same problems of serial ordering, even down to the temporal co-ordination of muscular contractions in such a movement as reaching and grasping. (121–2)

It is tempting to search for linguistic units which appear appropriate candidates for the neurolinguistic program. Among the most likely have been the *tone-unit* or *tone-group* (e.g. Halliday 1963). This unit is defined as a stretch of speech about six or seven syllables in length, usually bounded by pauses, and including one prominent syllable, which carries the major pitch movement of the tone-group. The nucleus (or prominent syllable) is normally located near the end of the tone-group and specifies the main intonational characteristics of the group. An example is the utterance 'That's a *'house*' (where ' = rising pitch), the nuclear pitch movement here signifying a questioning intonation which invites an answer such as 'yes' or 'no'.

The main evidence for postulating the tone group as a basic programming unit comes from two main sources; investigations into the location of pauses during speech (see later, chapter 3) and studies of breakdowns in the normal planning-and-execution process such as occur during slips of the tongue. The location of pauses in spontaneous speech was studied in an experiment carried out by Boomer (1965). He found that hesitations tended to occur near the beginnings of 'phonemic clauses' (equivalent to tone-groups), rather than be randomly distributed throughout the clauses. He reasoned that this was evidence for speech being encoded in terms of units larger than the word—the argument being that if the word were the basic unit, hesitations would be more likely to occur before those words with high information content, such as the lexical items carrying the nuclear pitch prominence. This in fact was not the case, so the experiment argued strongly for a phonemic clause rather than a word as the basic encoding unit (Boomer 1965, 156; see also Rochester 1973 for a review of similar experiments). It is interesting to note in this connection that many stutterers retain appropriate intonation patterns although manifesting disfluency features at the word level (see chapter 7).

Evidence for the tone-group as the basic organizational unit in the neuro-linguistic program has come also from studies of slips of the tongue (see the collection of representative articles in Fromkin 1973). In a study of tongue slips which occurred during a wide range of natural speech varieties, Boomer and Laver (1968) noted that the occurrence of these slips was not random but obeyed certain relatively well-defined structural principles. Most slips were 'anticipatory', i.e. the cause or origin of the slip typically occurred later in the speech utterance than the slip itself. Thus in the utterance 'But those frunds . . . funds have been frozen' (an example from Boomer and Laver 1968, 2), the tongue-slip 'frunds' occurs as a result of interference with the word 'frozen' appearing later in the utterance, and is immediately corrected by the speaker. It was found that the origin or cause of such anticipatory slips is typically the tonic (nuclear) word of the tone-group in which it occurs. The authors conclude:

> The fact that the span of interference in a slip is usually within one tone-group suggests that this unit is not simply a linguistic construct, but can plausibly be assumed to have behavioural properties as well. In our view, the tone-group is handled in the central nervous system as a unitary behavioural act, and the neural correlates of the separate elements are assembled and partially activated, or 'primed', before the performance of the utterance begins. This state of affairs whereby target and origin are simultaneously represented in an interim assembly maximizes the likelihood of interaction between them. This hypothesis also accounts for the observed fact that interactions across tone-group boundaries are fairly rare. (8–9)

The unitary nature of the tone-group provides further evidence for this unit as the basis for the neurolinguistic program.

It seems plausible, then, that the neurolinguistic program is organized by the central nervous system in terms of a unit the size of a tone-group. One would need to postulate also that the program is formulated in accordance with the semantic, syntactic and phonological rules of the language, and that this formulation requires the involvement of some sort of storage-and-retrieval system for linguistic items. As far as the semantic content of the program is concerned, this is probably selected from some sort of lexical storage system. Evidence from slips of the tongue such as 'sleast' (reported by Laver 1970), where there seems to be a confusion between 'least' and 'slightest', suggests that more lexical items are 'activated' or 'primed' than are ultimately selected for the neurolinguistic program. As Lashley (1951) points out, 'There are indications that, prior to the internal or covert enunciation of the sentence, an aggregate of word units is partially activated or readied' (155). We can hypothesize that some sort of monitoring takes place during the lexical selection process, in which a number of competing items will be compared for suitability in expressing the original idea. (As we shall see in chapter 7, this selection process is probably more complex for those stutterers who use strategies of word avoidance.) The coarseness of the monitoring process, incidentally, may depend on the time at the individual's disposal. If he is under time pressure, presumably the monitoring process may be more cursory. Thus, one would probably expect more lexical slips to occur in rapid, hurried speech than in slow, deliberate articulation. Likewise, the stutterer exhibits more pathological disfluencies the faster he talks (see chapter 7).

The procedures involved in selecting the appropriate item from the lexical store can be regarded as a problem in information-retrieval (see Laver 1970). Some sort of addressing system is necessary in the selection process, and factors such as associative lexical indices, and rhythm-and-stress patterns (see Brown and McNeill 1966; Laver 1970) obviously play an important role. We can gain some insight into the relative importance of these different indexing processes by studying the speech output of some aphasic patients with word-finding difficulties (see chapter 3 below, and Luria 1973).

The formulation of the neurolinguistic program at the syntactic level may involve similar procedures to those at the lexical level. One can postulate a sort of grammatical storage system containing the syntactic rules of the language, and a monitoring system assessing the suitability of the relevant syntactic construction for the expression of the original idea. There is obviously a close relationship between the selection of the syntactic construction and the lexical and phonological items in the planning process. Some investigators (e.g. Fromkin 1971) have suggested that the syntactic structure for the tone-group with its appropriate intonation and stress characteristics is specified in the programming stage prior to the selection of words from the lexical store. She hypothesizes a number of ordered stages in the generation of an utterance which may be summarized as follows:

Stage 1: generation of a 'meaning' or 'idea' to be conveyed
Stage 2: specification of the syntactic structure of the 'meaning', with semantic features associated with parts of the syntactic structure
Stage 3: generation of an appropriate intonation contour for the tone-group with the placement of primary (nuclear) stress
Stage 4: selection of words from the lexicon

Further stages are proposed which specify certain morphophonemic constraints imposed on the generation of the utterance, and finally the transmission of motor commands to speech muscles and the resulting speech activity.

An important requirement of the neurolinguistic program-planning system is that it ensures the smooth transition from one tone-group to the next. One could assume that there is some sort of sequential ordering device in the planning system to ensure that once a program has been executed, the next program in line is triggered. This would imply that for the normal speaker, a following program is being generated while the previous one is being executed by the speech organs. One can hypothesize also that a further requirement is that the neural traces of the program persist in some sort of short-term memory even after its motor execution.

Most of the above remarks can only be speculative in the absence of any direct objective experimental data on neural processes during speech encoding. It may be, for example, that the basic neurolinguistic program does not correspond to any linguistic concept such as the tone-group. Also, it is conceivable that the syntactic and semantic characteristics of the program are specified simultaneously rather than sequentially as has been suggested above. The definitive answer to such questions must await further research. The model remains, however, useful as a perspective in discussing pathological disorders where normal neurolinguistic functions are impaired.

A little more accessible to experimental investigation, however, is the question as to what are the *minimal* neural elements used in the assembly of the neuro-linguistic program. The two favoured linguistic candidates for these minimal units have been the phoneme and the syllable. To support the claim that the phoneme is the minimal element in the neurolinguistic program, various investi-gators (e.g. Liberman *et al.* 1967, 83; Harris *et al.* 1965; Öhman 1966) have used the technique of electromyography in an attempt to specify 'invariant' motor commands to articulatory organs such as the lips and velum, associated with the articulatory manifestations of any given phoneme. The EMG signals supposedly demonstrated the considerable degree of constancy in the motor commands issued to the muscles which accompany each phoneme. It is well known, however, that the acoustic and articulatory correlates of any given phoneme vary according to the context in which it appears. The authors of phoneme-based models would consider this peripheral variability to be due to factors such as mechanical and physiological constraints inherent in the speech structures, such as the mass and inertia of individual speech organs, as well as temporal overlapping in the neural signals for successive phonemes (MacNeilage 1970).

Evidence in support of the syllable as the minimal encoding unit has come also from electromyographic investigation. In a study of labial articulation by Fromkin (1968), evidence was offered to suggest that EMG readings for [p] and [b] differ according to whether these sounds are in initial or final position in the syllable, although there was some evidence of invariant neural commands for the phonemes in either of the two positions. Fromkin used this evidence to suggest that speech may be organized in terms of the syllable rather than the phoneme as the basic neural unit in the neurolinguistic program. The motor commands to phonemes would then be regarded as having neural invariance only in terms of their organiza-tion within the syllable. Further support for the syllable as the likely basic unit has come from the tongue-slip data (see in particular Fromkin 1971, Nooteboom 1969, Boomer and Laver 1968), Nooteboom (1969) for example, points out that 'the distance between origin and target does not generally exceed seven syllables . . . [and] since we know that the short memory span of man may contain about seven units at a time we might interpret our findings as an argument for the syllable to be a unit in the phonemic programming system.'

Rather than trying to postulate neural invariances corresponding to particular linguistic categories such as phoneme or syllable, MacNeilage (1970) proposes what might be called 'a target theory of speech production'. The basic premise of this theory is that 'speech is controlled, in part, by the specification of targets in an internalized space co-ordinate system' (189). The control of speech is said to be analogous to that of other human activities and that concepts taken from theories of general behaviour are applicable to speech. One of these concepts is the theory of 'motor equivalence' which accounts for 'a variability of specific muscular responses with circumstance in such a way as to produce a single result' (Hebb 1949, 153, cited by MacNeilage 1970). Thus a certain end result or target (such as opening a door, or making a particular speech articulation) remains the same but the detailed motor behaviour involved in reaching the goal can be variable (Mac-Neilage 1970, 186). For example in the two utterances 'eat' [i:t] and 'art' [a:t] the articulatory target position for [t] (namely lingual-palatal contact in the alveolar region and along the sides of the upper palate) is similar, although the positions of the articulatory organs for the initial vowels is quite different—in the first case the tongue is raised forwards and upwards close to the hard palate while in the second case the tongue is lying relatively flat in the oral cavity and the mandible is lowered. It seems to us that a target-based theory of speech production is quite plausible, although, in keeping with the emphasis on the dynamic aspects of the program-planning function, we would prefer to postulate the basic neural elements as corresponding to target *movements* or *gestures*. It is then necessary to show how the achievement of these target movements is controlled during speech production. This will be discussed below in the section on the monitoring function. First some features of the motor regulator and myodynamic execution system will be outlined.

Motor regulator function

As mentioned above, the motor regulator function is concerned with the specification of the output of the neurolinguistic program-planning stage in terms of sequences of motor commands to the speech muscles. We would postulate that the input to the regulator consists of both motor and sensory correlates of the articulatory target movements, and that the target movements are plotted with reference to an internalized spatial coordinate system of the vocal tract. Lashley (1951) recognizes the importance of an internalized spatial representation of the axes of the body during the maintenance of posture: 'This postural system is based on excitations from proprioceptors. The distance receptors impose an additional set of space coordinates upon the postural system, which in turn continually modifies the coordinates of the distance receptors. The dropped cat rights itself, if either the eyes or the vestibular senses are intact, but not in the absense of both' (190). It is plausible that such a space coordinate system exists for the vocal tract and serves as a sort of blueprint on which target movements are plotted in the motor regulator system. Because of the close association between motor activity and sensory information contributing to this internalized representation, any motor target specification will necessarily also incorporate an appropriate sensory schema of the vocal organs. The motor specifications of the target movement will include such factors as which articulatory organs are involved, which muscles or groups of muscles are to contract, the degree of force of contraction, the velocity of articulatory movement, and at a more microscopic level, which motor units in particular muscles should be activated and what sort of motor-unit firing is required. These motor correlates or specifications can be regarded collectively as constituting a *motor schema* for particular articulatory target movements. An appropriate *sensory schema* will also be specified. This will include details of the sensory consequences of the intended target movement such as the firing characteristics of particular proprioceptive and tactile receptor organs, which signal details of the location and pressure of contact between articulatory organs, and the relevant positions, speed and direction of movement of these organs. It seems plausible also that as part of the *sensory schema* the auditory consequences of the target movement, in terms of specific patterns of neural firing in the vestibulocochlear nerve, are also specified.

The motor and sensory schemata of the target movements are presumably organized not only with reference to the hypothesized spatial coordinate system of the vocal organs but also with reference to some sort of temporal 'grid' or 'pacemaker'. A number of researchers have speculated as to the neural correlates of this temporal 'organizing principle' (e.g. Lenneberg 1967, Bernstein 1967) and suggest that its basis is to be found in electroencephalographic rhythms recorded from various parts of the brain (see Brazier 1960). Lenneberg and Bernstein both mention an identifiable rhythm of 7 cycles per sec. We can assume that this frequency corresponds closely to the rate of articulation of successive target movements during the speech production process.

Myodynamic execution function

At the myodynamic execution stage in the generation of a speech utterance, the speech organs respond to the motor commands issued from the motor regulator system and move according to the appropriate motor schemata. Recent experimental phonetic research using techniques such as cinefluorography, electromyography and electropalatography has given us a much better understanding of the dynamics of articulatory activity and the sorts of constraints imposed on this activity by inherent physiological properties of the speech system (for reviews of such work see Harris 1974; MacNeilage 1972; Kim 1971; Hardcastle 1974, 1976). The constraints arise both from the transmission of motor impulses and the mechanics of muscular contraction. It is clear that the motor regulator has knowledge of such constraints and is able to modify motor commands appropriately. Compensation must be made in advance for different phonetic contexts, for example, so that articulatory organs are free to move in a continuous parametric fashion (see chapter 3).

Constraints involving the transmission of neural impulses are related to such biological factors as the diameter of the axon and composition of the myelin sheath. Also, the time taken for a neural impulse to reach a muscle is related to the length of the nerve fibre and the number of synapses traversed before reaching the muscle. The length of the motor pathway for a particular cranial nerve has interesting implications for the temporal coordination of such muscular systems as those of the tongue and the larynx, where the overall lengths of the motor nerves supplying these organs are different. As Lenneberg (1967) points out,

> the anatomy of the nerves suggests that innervation time for intrinsic laryngeal muscles may easily be up to 30 msec. longer than innervation time for muscles in and around the oral cavity. Considering now that some articulatory events may last as short a period as 20 msec., it becomes a reasonable assumption that the firing order in the brain stem may at times be different from the order of events occurring at the periphery. (96)

Although Lenneberg's ideas are interesting, one cannot place too much reliance on his methods of arriving at the figure of 30 msec. Short of actually isolating a particular nerve fibre in a living person and measuring the time taken for an impulse to be transmitted along its length, the figure mentioned by Lenneberg must remain speculative. Besides, this difference would only be relevant if the two motor fibres measured were identical in diameter, sheath composition etc. This is extremely difficult to ascertain in a typical cranial 'mixed' nerve which consists of a very large number of sensory and motor fibres of different diameters.

Other constraints on the myodynamic execution system arise from the mechanics of muscular contraction. For example, the degree of force developed by a muscle and the time taken to achieve this force in tetanic contraction will depend on a number of factors including mechanical properties of the muscle such as its mass, elasticity, and inertia, the number of motor units active at any one time, the frequency of successive activations within motor units, and the mechanical properties of an imposed load (see Roberts 1966). There must be some elements in the speech system which can make necessary compensations for these muscular constraints to control the precisely timed articulatory movements. Bernstein (1967), when discussing the lack of one-to-one correspondence between motor commands and actions produced at various junctures, says, 'It is clear that organisms, whose only channels of operation upon the surrounding world are commands given to their muscles, can achieve controlled movements serving a particular purpose only by means of continuous monitoring and control achieved by the participation of the sense organs' (146). A description of the various functions of monitoring systems used in the planning and execution of speech utterances will comprise the final section of this chapter.

Monitoring function

It is clear that some form of monitoring is used in the speech production process; to verify this, one need only consider the fact that we frequently detect and correct slips of the tongue. We have speculated above that monitoring can exist at all stages in the speech generation process; for example during the formulation of the neurolinguistic program to check for suitability in expressing the underlying idea or intention, and during the myodynamic execution process to assess the accuracy of an ongoing target movement against the motor and sensory schema

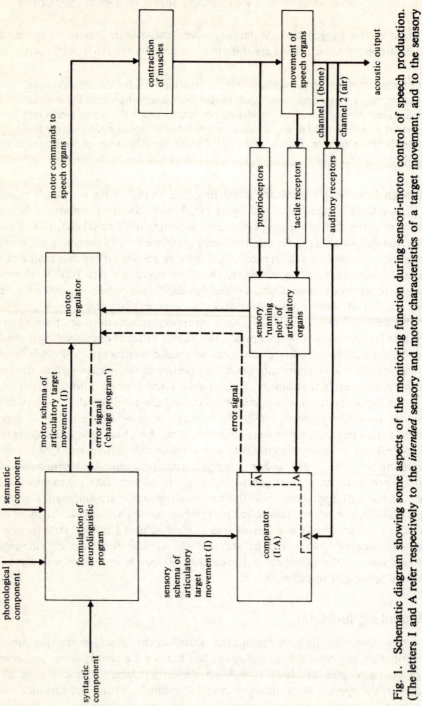

Fig. 1. Schematic diagram showing some aspects of the monitoring function during sensori-motor control of speech production. (The letters I and A refer respectively to the *intended* sensory and motor characteristics of a target movement, and to the sensory characteristics that *actually* obtain in the speech and hearing apparatus at a given time)

for that movement. We know relatively more about the latter, more peripheral type of monitoring and are in a position to speculate about its possible role during ongoing speech production.

We can hypothesize that a monitoring system ensures that the target movements are accurately executed and, when they are not, it directs the motor regulator or the program-planning system to take appropriate steps to correct the error. The monitoring system probably consists of the following basic processes: an *input* comprising the motor commands to the speech muscles, *feedback* of afferent information from sensory receptor organs situated in the oral mucosa, the speech muscles and the inner ear, *comparison* of the sensory information with the idealized target schema, and appropriate *modification* of motor commands in the motor regulator system. These different processes in the monitoring system are illustrated schematically in Fig. 1, and are discussed more fully below.

It can be seen from the diagram how motor commands are issued to the muscles of the speech organs, which move under the influence of muscular contraction and so produce speech sounds. There are three main sensory channels to provide feedback for the comparator and motor regulator systems; a *tactile* feedback channel, from mechanoreceptors situated mainly in the oral mucosa conveying information concerning the precise location, the pressure and the timing of contacts between articulatory structures; a *proprioceptive* feedback channel from muscle spindles, tendon organs and joint receptors in the speech muscles and joints, conveying information such as the length of a muscle fibre, degree of stretch of the fibre, and rate of change of muscle length; and an *auditory* feedback channel from hair-cells in the Organ of Corti of the inner ear conveying information about acoustic characteristics of the sound resulting from articulatory movements. (As seen in Fig. 1, the acoustic feedback is conducted via two channels representing the acoustic pathways to the ear through the air and through the body tissues and bones.)

As we saw above, one important function of the feedback of detailed sensory information from these three channels is that it enables the central processing units to build up an internal space coordinate system of the oral tract to serve as a blueprint on which the target schemata are plotted. Closely related to their functions in providing a detailed space coordinate system of the vocal tract is the role played by the feedback mechanisms in the ongoing control of articulation. The feedback channels are here used to provide a continuous running 'plot' of the situation that actually obtains at the periphery of the body to be compared with the idealized target movements. For both the tactile and auditory systems, sensory information is sent after the event only, i.e. after contact is made between articulatory structures or after speech sound waves have impinged upon the eardrum. Because of the special properties of the proprioceptive system, however, particularly that part of the system comprising muscle spindles and their innervation, information can be sent not only after the event but also *during* the articulatory movement while muscles are contracting. The potential for such 'in-process' monitoring illustrates the prodigious versatility of the muscle spindle system, and many investigators (e.g. MacNeilage 1970, 1972; Bowman 1971; Smith and

Lee 1972) have begun to recognize the possibilities of feedback control by muscle spindles during speech. We felt that, in view of this increasing interest in the potential role of the muscle spindle in monitoring ongoing speech production, a relatively detailed account of the main physiological characteristics of the spindle would be useful at this point.

Muscle spindles have been located in the muscles of all speech organs and consist basically of small receptor organs enclosed in spindle-shaped connective-tissue sheaths running parallel with the main (extrafusal) fibres of the muscle (see Fig. 2 and the detailed descriptions of muscle spindles in Matthews 1964,

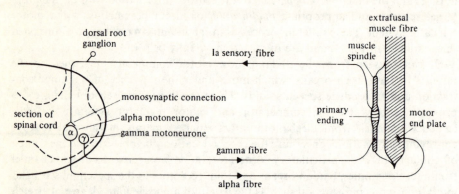

Fig. 2.   Diagram showing some of the main characteristics of the muscle spindle system

1972; Cooper 1960; Bowman 1971). Because of their attachments to muscle fibres, any change in length of the muscle as a whole will also affect the spindles. Thus stretch on the main muscle, due for example, to contradiction of an antagonistic muscle will result in stretch on the spindle. Special receptor organs called primary endings (or annulospiral endings) within the muscle spindles respond directly to these mechanical changes in the spindle: the greater the degree of stretch the higher the frequency of neural discharge in the primary endings. The discharge in the primary endings of muscle spindles will thus accurately reflect the length of the muscle as a whole: when the muscle is stretched the discharge will have a higher frequency than when the muscle is shortened. Not only, however, do primary endings respond to the degree of stretch on the spindle, they respond also to the *rate of change* of stretch. This dynamic property of the primary ending discharge has possible important implications for the control of speech production as it is one way in which the central nervous system can obtain *predictive* information about the progress of a particular target movement (see below).

The afferent fibres from primary endings in muscle spindles (so-called Ia fibres) project to the cerebral cortex via several synaptic junctions and are thought by some investigators (e.g. Eccles 1973, 119) to give important information concerning the movement and position of a bodily structure. As Eccles puts it (119) 'In fact their [i.e. group Ia fibres] principal function may be to signal to the cerebral cortex the progress of the movement that it has just previously programmed.'

We would maintain that the discharge from primary fibres of muscle spindles in the speech organs provide an essential part of the sensory schema for a target movement as well as providing ongoing information concerning the length of the muscles. ·

Another characteristic of the muscle spindle which has attracted a great deal of attention is its role as an automatic regulator of body posture. Some investigators have claimed that this function is similar to that of a self-regulating system or servo mechanism (e.g. Merton 1953). This function of the muscle spindle depends on the fact that the Ia afferent fibres make monosynaptic connections with motoneurones supplying the muscle within which the spindle is situated. This activation of the main motoneurones (alpha (a) fibres) causes the muscle to contract reflexly, so shortening the length of individual fibres, which in turn reduces the firing frequency in the primary endings. This mechanism is the basis of the so-called stretch reflex loop, which can be seen clearly in its rudimentary form in the familiar knee jerk. It is probable that a similar mechanism to that outlined above occurs in the cranial nerve system, although most investigations have been carried out so far with reference to reflex loops in the spinal system.

The servo mechanism function of the spindle system in maintaining a constant muscle length is an extremely elegant piece of biological engineering, and is made even more so by the addition of an extra facility for 'biasing' the servo mechanism. To understand how this biasing is carried out it is necessary to consider more closely the structure of the spindle. In addition to the main sensory receptor (the primary ending) each spindle contains a number of thin muscle fibres which run parallel with the main extrafusal fibres of the muscle. These small (intrafusal) fibres have separate innervation from the main extrafusal fibres and their contraction causes a powerful excitation of the primary endings, the degree of excitation depending on the degree of tension exerted by the intrafusal fibres. This primary ending discharge will in turn cause monosynaptic firing of the alpha motoneurones to the extrafusal muscle fibres which contract and so reduce the firing from the primary endings in the spindle. Because the activity of the spindle reflex loop can be altered according to activity of the gamma motor fibres, the gamma system is said to bias the servo loop mechanism.

The potential implications of the gamma loop control of the muscle spindle for the control of speech production has been recognized by a number of investigators (notably MacNeilage 1970). The theory depends on the fact that a motor command can be sent along the gamma system appropriate for the muscle as a whole to achieve a desired length. This length will be automatically achieved irrespective of the length of the muscle at the beginning of the gamma activity, by the operation of the normal spindle reflex loop. As Milner (1970) says 'with the servo mechanism, each value of the output from the higher-level control corresponds not to a certain muscle contraction but to a particular position of the muscle, independent of load, and this relationship greatly simplifies the problem of making accurate movements' (67). The 'accurate movements' may be, for example, articulatory movements towards the alveolar ridge for a stop such as [t] in two different environments [aːt] ('art') and [iːt] ('eat').

This theory of gamma-loop activity assumes that a movement is initiated by appropriate neural firing along the gamma fibres. Some investigators had suggested that discharge of gamma motoneurones may indeed precede that of alpha moto-neurones in the same muscle (e.g. Cooper 1960; Matthews 1964); however, this view has recently been challenged (see Vallbo 1971, cited by Eccles 1973). Eccles (1973) summarizes the function of the alpha-gamma motor complex as follows:

> in voluntary movement . . . impulses excite both α and γ motoneurones (*coactivation*), the whole α-γ complex being put into action in an approximately synchronous manner. The α motoneurones are excited to discharge impulses and so bring about the muscle contraction. At about the same time the motoneurones discharge, so exciting the muscle spindles and setting the loop in operation. Because of the time involved in traversing the γ loop, the α motoneurone discharge so generated by the Ia impulses would not occur until after the muscle had started to contract. It thus occurs at just the right time for the onset of the servo mechanism control. (117)

These observations were made with specific reference to the spinal system. It seems plausible that the same applies to the cranial nerve system during speech activity.

The spindle, then, by means of the primary ending discharge can provide moment-to-moment information on the length of the muscle and the rate of change of length. By providing information on the rate of change of length, it is plausible that the spindle can provide predictive data, for example on the length that the muscle will achieve after a given period of time. The spindle also plays an important role as a servo mechanism making automatic compensations for external changes imposed on the muscle.

The main characteristics of the three main sensory feedback channels, pro-prioceptive, tactile and auditory, are slightly different and this means that their respective roles in the monitoring of speech articulation also differs. The pro-prioceptive system, for example, operates through larger-diameter nerve fibres, which means that the conduction velocity of neural impulses will be extremely high—higher, for example, than the smaller fibres in the tactile system. This means the proprioceptive system is very fast-acting, an essential requirement, incidentally, for use in the control of speech production. The auditory system which relies on the transmission of sound through the air and the vibration of bones in the skull is slower-acting than either of the other two systems. In chapter 7 we shall be dis-cussing the role of auditory feedback in stuttering.

One can speculate that the different sorts of sensory feedback are exploited at different stages in the execution of an articulatory target movement—the pro-prioceptive system coming into operation during the movement itself, the tactile system operating after contact is made between articulatory structures, and the auditory system operating after the production of sounds. It is plausible also that a given type of sensory feedback may vary in its importance depending on the category of articulation involved. Thus tactile feedback will be primarily important for those types of articulations involving contact between speech organs, e.g.

between tongue and palate; auditory feedback may be primarily important for vowel articulation, particularly open vowels which involve very little contact between articulatory structures, and also for monitoring of prosodic features such as pitch, stress and duration variations. Proprioceptive feedback is probably important for all articulatory activities where precise positioning of the speech organs is necessary, e.g. during production of 'grooved' fricatives [s], [ʃ], and most vowels.

The following table summarizes the main characteristics of the three feedback systems and their hypothesized roles in speech production.

Characteristics of the main feedback systems used in the control of speech

	Tactile	Proprioceptive	Auditory
Type of sensory receptors	(1) 'free' endings (2) 'complex' endings (e.g. Krause end-bulbs, Meissner corpuscles)	(1) muscle spindles (2) Golgi tendon organs (3) joint receptors	hair cells in Organ of Corti
Distribution of receptors	(1) superficial layers of oral mucosa (2) lamina propria, particularly deeper layers	(1) all speech muscles (2) tendons (3) capsules of joints	Organ of Corti in cochlea
Information sent to CNS	(1) and (2) { (a) localization of contact (b) pressure of contact (c) direction of movement (d) onset time of contact	(1) { (a) length of muscle fibre (b) velocity of stretch (c) direction of movement of muscle (2) { change of stretch on tendon by muscular contraction etc. (3) { (a) rate of joint movement (b) direction of joint movement (c) extent of joint movement	(a) intensity (b) frequency (c) direction of sounds (d) periodicity (e) duration

	Tactile	Proprioceptive	Auditory
Main features of the feedback systems	(a) slower-acting than proprioceptive because (i) multisynaptic (ii) afferent fibres smaller	(a) fast-acting because (i) monosynaptic (ii) spindle afferent fibres largest in body	(a) slower-acting than tactile and proprioceptive because transmission of sound through air (for air conduction)
	(b) spatial projection of peripheral receptive surface preserved in sensory cortex and cerebellum	(b) predictive information important for servo operation	(b) projection on auditory cortex preserves spatial characteristics of basilar membrane, also projections to other areas
	(c) probably transmits information *after* the event	(c) speech target 'invariance' by means of 'follow-up length servo' operation of gamma loop system	(c) supplies information *after* the event
	(d) important for speech movements involving contact between articulators e.g. [t], [i] etc.	(d) provides information *during* the event	(d) important for open and back vowels (e.g. [a], [o])
		(e) important for all articulations requiring precise positioning of articulatory structures	(e) important for prosodic features such as pitch, duration, stress

It remains to be shown how the monitoring of target movements takes place using the sensory information provided by the feedback channels. The process is schematized in Fig. 1 (p. 16). The sensory schema for an *intended* target articulation (I) is fed into a comparator unit together with sensory feedback information from the periphery of the speech organs indicating the *actual* position the vocal organs are adopting at any given time (A). This sensory feedback information corresponds to the continuous 'running plot' mentioned above (p. 17). The difference between the intended goal I and the actual position A reached by the articulators is calculated by the comparator in terms of what is usually called an 'error signal' (see Fairbanks 1954). Thus at any given time the error signal gives a measure of the amount by which the target articulation has not yet been reached by the speech organs. If the error signal equals zero then the goal I will equal A and the *next* element of the program (presumably the next target movement) is 'triggered off' and proceeds to the myodynamic execution stage. If, however, the error signal does not equal zero it provides data which enables the motor commands to the muscles (i.e. the motor schema of the target movement) to be adjusted so as to bring the error signal closer to zero.

This adjustment probably takes place at the motor regulator into which both the error signal and the motor schema are fed. The motor commands to the muscles are modified until the error signal is reduced. This closed-loop process continues until the motor commands are modified so that the output equals the intended target. It is probable, however, that the output will not *always* exactly equal the intended target. Presumably, a certain amount of error signal is permitted before any correctional activities take place. It is probable also that some target movements, in fact often whole sequences of target movements may be executed without any closed-loop feedback involvement, the only monitoring occurring after a stretch of speech and involving the auditory feedback channel. Other target movements, for example those involving precise tongue configurations such as during [s], may rely considerably on the closed-loop feedback monitoring for the accuracy of their production.

Some investigators (e.g. Lashley 1951) have suggested that closed-loop systems such as the one outlined above involve a certain amount of time for the neural impulses to travel round the feedback circuit, and because of this time-lag it would not be possible for such systems to control fast, accurate movements. For this reason Lashley postulates that an effector mechanism can be 'preset' or 'primed' to discharge at a given intensity or for a given duration, independent of any sensory controls. We would agree that some sequences of target movements can be 'triggered off as a whole' in this way, but we would suggest that the characteristics of the feedback circuits used in speech production make them perhaps more suitable for closed-loop control than Lashley suggests. It is not known, for example, just how fast proprioceptive feedback can operate in the cranial system; one could assume that it would be at least as fast as the eye-blink reflex (see Kugelberg 1952 and Rushworth 1966) measured at 12–15 msec. or less. It would seem also that, because of the shorter distances involved, the feedback of afferent information and subsequent motor commands via the large-diameter fibres in the cranial nerve (i.e. those supplying the primary endings of muscle spindles and tactile receptors) would be considerably faster than would be the case with reflex arcs associated with fast movements of the hand.

However, even assuming there were no feedback mechanisms fast enough to provide ongoing control, it is not necessary that the target movement be completed before afferent information is sent back to the planning unit. In fact, it seems plausible that the regulator and planning systems can extrapolate into the future, and so predict the position that the articulatory organs will attain after a specific interval of time. We have seen above how the muscle spindle is capable of providing 'predictive' information about the behaviour of a muscle, thus allowing compensation in advance by the regulator system. Consequently, it may not be necessary for each stage of the planning function (i.e. each target movement) to wait until the error signal of the previous stage equals zero. As Fairbanks (1954) says,

The advancement of the storage component to the next control point is not
necessarily delayed until the actual moment when a condition of zero error signal

obtains. It can be triggered in advance of that time by an amount, let us say, equal to the relevant time constants. By this means, over suitable channels, a new input can be started on its way towards the effector before the previous control point has been reached, so that it will arrive there at an appropriate anticipated time. (137)

The smooth triggering of successive target movements is an important requirement for normal fluent speech. To facilitate such smooth transition it is necessary for the motor regulator to 'scan ahead' to at least the next target movement in line and make appropriate modifications to the current target movement being processed. This implies that the motor regulator must be in constant touch with details of the current neurolinguistic program being processed at any given time. It is only by maintaining such constant surveillance that the motor regulator can ensure that the speech organs move in a parallel fashion and so enable coarticulation to occur freely (see chapter 3). Breakdown in the smooth transition between successive elements in the neurolinguistic program and between successive programs themselves is seen as the basis for a number of different types of pathological disfluencies (see for example the efferent motor aphasia described by Luria 1973).

The precise anatomical and physiological correlates of those functions in the speech-generation process which involve the central nervous system, i.e. the ideation, neurolinguistic program planning, motor regulation and monitoring functions, are at present unknown. We know however that breakdowns can occur involving any of these neural functions as well as the myodynamic execution function, and such breakdowns may be manifested by relatively specific speech abnormalities. For example, a disorder involving the ideation stage may be manifested by general aspontaneity of speech, and inability to retain the original idea or intention long enough to program and execute an appropriate neurolinguistic plan. Luria describes 'aspontaneity of speech' as one of the main characteristics of frontal lobe lesions (1973, 319). Disorders can also occur which involve different stages of the program-planning function. The process of selection of items from the lexical store may be impaired in patients and is called anomia, a general disability to name objects correctly. The temporal sequencing of elements in the program can also be altered as in patients with dyspraxia of speech (one of the manifestations of Luria's efferent motor aphasia) (see discussion in chapter 8). This disorder may be manifested by difficulties in triggering off successive target movements, as was seen above, but also by general problems in formulating appropriate neurolinguistic plans for expression of the initial idea, although more automatic non-speech activities of the articulatory organs such as swallowing or chewing may be carried out quite normally. Abnormalities can also occur in the monitoring function, e.g. in the feedback of tactile and proprioceptive information to the area of the cerebral cortex just posterior to the central fissure of Rolando (as in Luria's (1973) afferent motor aphasia) and in the feedback of acoustic information to the so-called auditory (temporal) cortex (as in predominantly receptive aphasia). The integration and processing of much of the feedback data probably takes place in regions such as the brain stem and in the cerebellum, and lesions in these areas can lead to relatively inaccurate articulatory target movements, particularly when they involve precise configuration and positioning of articulatory organs as in the fricatives [s] and [ʃ].

Disorders can also occur involving the myodynamic execution function. In most of these cases either the transmission pathways of neural impulses supplying the speech organs are impaired (as for example in most of the dysarthrias) or there is some organic disability in the speech organ itself (e.g. cleft-palate, macroglossia, malocclusion). In these cases, central planning processes are normally intact, the disorder residing predominantly at the more automatic articulatory level.

This chapter, then, has been an attempt to provide a suitable theoretical framework within which to describe normal and pathological speech. The main characteristics of the proposed model have been described in terms of a central planning function (involving the ideation and neurolinguistic program-planning stages), an executive function (involving the motor regulation and motor execution stages), and a monitoring function, operating at various stages in the speech-generation process and utilizing a variety of sensory feedback channels. It is important to separate the three main functions—planning, execution and monitoring—in any consideration of disordered speech, as these three functions can be differentially affected under various pathological conditions.

In the latter part of this volume we shall discuss more specifically how the three main functions can be affected in conditions of stuttering and cluttering, and in other speech and language disorders manifesting disfluencies.

3

Some speech variables
involved in an evaluation of fluency

In chapter 1 some of the speech variables or indices used in the assessment of fluency were outlined, and we saw how these indices were generally related to the temporal ordering (transition smoothness) of speech events at the output end of the encoding process. In this chapter we will begin by considering in more detail the concept of transition smoothness and then discuss under the headings of pausing, rhythmical patterning, and regulation of tempo some specific variables related to transition smoothness in both normal and pathological speech.

Transition smoothness

As discussed in chapter 1, transition smoothness operates at four levels—at the articulatory phonetic level, relating mainly to transitions between speech segments and syllables; at the grammatical level relating to transitions between syntactic units such as phrases, clauses and sentences; at the prosodic level, relating to transitions between rhythmical stress and intonation units such as tone-groups; and at the lexical/semantic level, relating to thematic elements in a discourse. At the articulatory phonetic level, lack of transition smoothness is manifested typically by prolongations and omissions of speech elements, and by repetitions of sound segments and syllables; at the grammatical level it is reflected mainly by the omission of grammatical 'linking' devices such as the coordinators 'and', 'but' etc.; and at the prosodic level lack of transition smoothness will primarily affect the relationships between adjacent prosodic units, such as tone-groups, and will be manifested typically by abnormal sequential patterning of intonation contours over a stretch of spontaneous connected speech. At the lexical/semantic level, transition smoothness may be impaired when inappropriate words are used or when ideas fail to follow a logical sequence in a discourse.

In discussing transition smoothness at the articulatory phonetic level it is convenient to consider the motor commands to speech muscles as being encoded in the CNS primarily in terms of idealized articulatory 'targets' or 'target movements' which may or may not correspond to linguistic units such as phonemes (cf. MacNeilage 1970). Although these motor commands may reflect idealized targets in terms of a specific configuration of articulatory organs at some early stage in the execution of the neurolinguistic program (see p. 9), the targets themselves are almost invariably not achieved exactly by the speech organs but are only approximated. As we saw in chapter 2 there are a number of plausible reasons for this, mainly arising from physiological constraints on the articulatory processes: mechano-inertial forces of different organs, overlapping motor commands for successive targets etc. In normal speech, the extent to which a given target is undershot or overshot will depend largely on such external factors as overall speed of utterance, those targets which precede or follow it, and prosodic features such as stress, rhythm and intonation. Normal speech production requires that transitions between successive targets be relatively smooth, and this sort of smooth transition can only be achieved by precise coordination between the three main speech physiological systems: the *supraglottal system*, consisting of articulatory organs in the vocal tract above the level of the glottis (soft palate, pharynx, tongue, mandible and lips), the *laryngeal system*, consisting of the cartilages of the larynx and the vocal cords, and the *subglottal system*, comprising the thoracic cage (enclosing the lungs), and the diaphragm. The participation of these three physiological systems in the coordination of normal speech articulation can be illustrated by considering, in a relatively detailed manner, a typical pronunciation of the word 'too' (/tu/), in the phrase 'too many people'. The detailed analysis of the pronunciation of this word will then serve as a background for the discussion which follows on what happens during a breakdown of transition smoothness as in the case of some pathologically disfluent speakers.

During the initial part of the articulation of 'too' the lower jaw (mandible) is raised slightly and the tongue moved foward and upwards in the mouth to make contact along the sides of the upper gums and palate, and across the alveolar ridge just posterior to the upper front teeth. This tongue contact makes an effective seal preventing air passing into or out of the mouth. The soft palate meanwhile is raised to close off the nasal cavity from the oral cavity and so prevent air passing out of the nose. The degree of muscular precision required to make the tongue contact is probably relatively crude. It is sufficient merely to maintain closure, a precise tongue configuration not being necessary. The situation is quite different for the articulation of a fricative sound such as the initial sound in 'Sue', where a precise configuration in the surface of the tongue, namely a narrow central groove, as well as precise positioning of the organ in the mouth is necessary to create fricative noise with the specific acoustic characteristics of this sound.

Simultaneously with the attainment of the tongue closure for the initial sound in 'too', the lips are slightly rounded and pushed forward. It is interesting to note that such lip movement is in no way part of the normal articulatory target specification of /t/ but is appropriate for the following vowel /u/. This is an example of anticipatory coarticulation where it is as if all motor commands for the components of target movements in an entire syllable are issued simultaneously at the onset of that syllable as long as they are non-contradictory (Kozhevnikov and Chistovich 1965). Such coarticulation occurs continually in speech and assists in the smooth transmission from sound to sound (for a detailed description of the sorts of coarticulation that typically occur in English, see Gimson, 1970).

At the level of the larynx, during the period of tongue closure, the space between the vocal cords (or glottis, as this space is sometimes called) is kept relatively wide by activity of the laryngeal abductor muscles to enable air to pass through from the lungs into the oral region. The tension in the vocal cord muscles and the width of the glottis are at this time not yet appropriate for voicing (i.e. vibration of the cords themselves) to occur, so air can flow relatively unimpeded through from the subglottal region under the influence of contraction of the thoracic cavity, e.g. by the activity of the intrinsic intercostal muscles and the so-called relaxation pressure (Ladefoged 1967). As the expelled air passes up through the glottis and into the supraglottal region, it encounters the obstruction caused by the tongue and soft palate, and air pressure builds up in the oral region. The air pressure there begins now to approximate the pressure below the glottis. Towards the end of the closure phase (i.e. while the tongue is maintaining contact with the palate), the larynx as a whole may be slightly raised, thus increasing even more the pressure above the glottis so that pressure above and below will be almost equalized.

At this point, the tip of the tongue is lowered suddenly and the build-up of pressure in the supralaryngeal region, which is now greater than atmospheric pressure, is released suddenly from the mouth as a puff of air. At the release also, the pressure in the supraglottal region suddenly becomes greatly reduced and air can flow easily from the subglottal to supraglottal regions. This creates a trans-glottal flow which is one of the conditions necessary for voicing (Van den Berg 1958). At the same time the glottis begins to narrow and the tension in the vocal cord muscles becomes appropriate for the voicing mode. However, because the conditions for voicing are not favourable immediately at the release of the tongue, due to the combined effect of factors such as inappropriate tension in the vocal cords and width of the glottis, voicing will not occur simultaneously with the release but will be delayed. This is not so in the case of the /d/ in the word 'do' where voicing will normally occur immediately at the release of the tongue. The temporal delay between the release of an articulatory organ (in this case, the tongue) and the onset of glottal pulsing for voicing is called the Voice Onset Time and has been suggested as an important feature in the classification of stop consonants in all languages (Lisker and Abramson 1964).

As the tongue tip is being released, the back part of the tongue is already rising towards the palate in anticipation of the vowel /u/, such that at the release there is only a very short delay before the tongue configuration appropriate for the vowel is achieved. The tongue is maintained in a fairly high, back position while the vowel sound is produced.

To summarize the above phonetic description, the precise coordination between the supraglottal, laryngeal and subglottal systems during the articulation of 'too' can be illustrated schematically as in Fig. 3 by means of a set of continuously varying parameters.

One can appreciate the enormous complexity of the articulatory coordination required for connected speech, where not only do a wide range of complex sounds occur (such as 'grooved' fricatives [s] and [ʃ], as in 'six' and 'shows' respectively), but there are added constraints imposed on the system because of prosodic features such as stress, intonation and rhythm operating over a whole stretch of speech, and affecting the interaction between all three physiological systems. This means

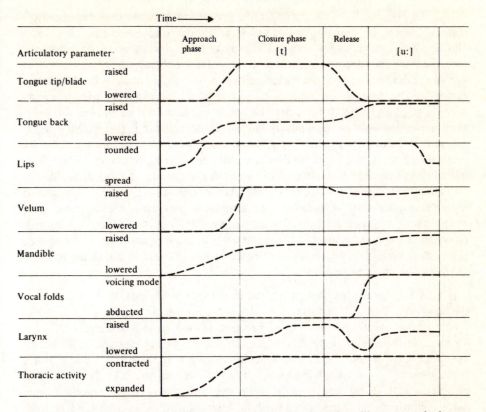

Fig. 3. Diagram showing a set of phonetic parameters used to illustrate articulatory activity during production of the word 'too' [tʰuː]

that, in pathological speech, there are many possible ways that the smooth coordination between adjacent sounds can break down.

It is convenient to consider the breakdown in coordination between the supraglottal, laryngeal and subglottal systems under two headings: breakdowns which occur at the motor speech level due, for example, to impairments in the neuromuscular characteristics of the articulatory and respiratory organs, and breakdowns which occur at the level of sensori-motor control due, for example, to malfunctioning of the sensory feedback control systems used in monitoring speech performance (see chapter 2). It is not proposed here to give a detailed description of all neuromuscular and sensori-motor pathologies that could impair normal articulatory coordination, but simply to indicate some ways this can happen, particularly in those disorders which manifest disfluencies.

At the motor speech level we will consider three situations where a breakdown in coordination can occur: first, when there is an abnormally high tension in the speech musculature; secondly, when the muscular tension is inadequate for the articulatory movement required; and thirdly, when there is a lack of balanced contraction between muscle groups which have opposing functions.

(*1*)   An abnormally high tension in the speech muscles has been suggested for some stutterers by many investigators (e.g. Lebrun and Boers-van Dijk 1973, Guitar 1975), and also for some of the dysarthrias, including ataxia (although here the muscular strength is relatively unpredictable, being sometimes too great and sometimes inadequate). Increased tension in articulatory muscles will frequently cause overshooting of articulatory targets so that, for example, fricatives may become stops and stop closures may be prolonged beyond their normal duration. Such a prolongation of articulatory closure could cause a higher buildup in air pressure in the oral cavity than is necessary and this may in turn result in difficulty in achieving the transglottal air flow necessary for voicing to occur. Difficulty in initiating voicing has been frequently noted for stutterers as have difficulties in transition from voiced to voiceless sounds. At the level of the glottis, also, increased muscular tension in the intrinsic laryngeal muscles may cause a complete closure of the glottis where a configuration appropriate for normal voicing is required. As we shall see later (chapter 7) a frequent manifestation of many stutterers' speech is hard blocking involving complete closure at the glottis and associated increase in tension of the laryngeal muscles.

(*2*)   When there is insufficient tension in the speech muscles, as for example in the so-called 'flaccid dysarthrias', the delicate coordinatory balance between the speech physiological systems can also be upset. If the hypoglossal nerve is affected, for example, the tension in the tongue muscles may not be appropriate for maintaining the closure necessary for a stop articulation such as in the initial sound in 'too'. If the closure is not maintained with sufficient strength to cause the buildup in pressure and the subsequent release of air, the distinction between voiceless stops (with aspiration) and voiced stops (without aspiration) may be difficult to achieve.

(*3*)   Another neuromuscular condition which can severely impair coordination between the three speech physiological systems is a lack of balanced contraction in muscle groups of specific speech organs. Simultaneous contraction of both protagonist and antagonist muscles has been noted in 'spastic dysarthria', particularly that associated with cerebral palsy. Darley, Aronson and Brown (1975) suggest that in many cerebral palsied speakers normal respiratory patterns are disrupted by inhalatory movements of the thoracic muscles being coincident with exhalatory movements of the abdominal muscles. This is known as 'reversed breathing' and results in a reduced vital capacity for those patients, leading to a more rapid breathing rate than normal. Lack of balanced contraction between protagonist and antagonist muscles has been noted also in the laryngeal musculature of some stutterers at the moment of the stuttering block (Freeman *et al.* 1975).

Disruption in sensory feedback control can also cause breakdowns in motor coordination between speech physiological systems, leading to a lack of smooth transitions between speech-sound segments and syllables. In chapter 2, characteristics of the three main sensory feedback channels—the auditory, tactile and proprioceptive—and their possible functions in monitoring speech productions were outlined. It was seen how sensory feedback can have reflexive or nonreflexive functions—the reflexive functions taking place below the level of the cortex, for example at the level of the lower neurone pool in the brain stem for the cranial nerve system and probably operating in much the same way as reflexive feedback loops in the spinal nerve system (such as the familiar knee jerk). Some investigators have suggested that for some stutterers there is an exaggeratedly high response in the mechanoreceptors of the larynx, reflexly triggering increased tension in the laryngeal muscles (Lebrun and Boers-van Dijk 1973). It is claimed that these mechanoreceptors can respond to a buildup in air pressure as would occur frequently in speech, as for example during the closure of stop consonants. The resulting abnormally high tension in the laryngeal muscles may explain the frequently cited observation that stuttering blocks occur far more frequently on initial consonants and stressed medial consonants than on final consonants (Van Riper 1971); also that blocks occur more often on consonants than vowels, as consonants are normally associated with relatively higher intra-oral pressure (see chapter 7).

The possible role of sensory feedback in facilitating the smooth transition between articulatory movements was discussed in chapter 2. It was seen how sensory feedback channels may signal to the Central Nervous System that one element of the neurolinguistic program has been completed, or at least that the motor commands appropriate for the movement have been sent out, and the next element can now be triggered. A disruption in this type of sensorimotor coordination may result after damage to the region at the foot of the third frontal convolution (Broca's area) in the dominant cortical hemisphere and may lead to the pathological condition which Luria (1973) calls efferent (or kinetic) motor aphasia. He characterizes this condition as a 'difficulty in switching from one articulation to another' and proceeds to exemplify:

the process of denervation of the preceding articuleme is profoundly disturbed, signs of *pathological inertia of an existing articulation* arise, and the smooth pronunciation of a polysyllabic word becomes impossible. In an attempt to pronounce the word 'mukha' the patient articulates the first (labial) syllable 'mu' properly, but cannot change to the next . . . syllable 'kha' and instead of the word required he can only say 'mu . . . m . . . m . . . mu . . . ma'. (185)

In their linguistic description of different types of aphasia, Jakobson and Halle (1956) regard Luria's efferent motor aphasia as primarily a 'combination' (in the temporal sense) disorder and list typical manifestations involving lack of transition smoothness such as difficulties using phoneme clusters and difficulties in transition from one syllable to another. The repetitions of syllables observed in some stutterers may conceivably be associated with some impairment in feedback, resulting in a momentary inability to inhibit already executed articulations and 'trigger' following ones.

So far we have considered transition smoothness at the articulatory phonetic level. However, the same general concept can be applied to transitions between grammatical structures and between prosodic units such as tone-groups, although the physiological and neurological conditioning factors for these phenomena may be quite different from those we have considered for the phonetic ones. At the syntactic grammatical level, lack of transition smoothness may be manifested by omission of grammatical linking devices such as coordinators 'and', 'but' etc. and subordinators 'who', 'which', 'what' etc. Omission of the linking conjunctions and other 'function' words have been mentioned as characteristics of certain types of expressive aphasia, particularly the motor efferent type described by Luria. The speech of such aphasics is frequently described as a 'telegraphic' style where 'there is no indication of grammatical coordination or subordination; there are few inflectional endings and almost all grammatical function words are missing' (Goodglass 1973, 185). Jakobson and Halle (1956) in their linguistic analysis of aphasic types see the 'telegraphic' style as another of the characteristics of contiguity disorders (in addition to lack of transition smoothness at the phonetic level) in the efferent motor aphasic (see above). Frequently, according to Goodglass, these patients use single words or short-phrase sentences in which the syntactic relationships are often obscure or are implied only by contiguity and sequence (see further discussion in chapter 8).

Transition smoothness at the level of prosodic features has not usually been considered in the speech pathology literature as a possible index of speech disfluency. However, as pointed out by Crystal (1975, ch. 1), interactions between adjacent tone-groups—for example modifications to the tonal characteristics of a given tone-group (direction of pitch movement on the nucleus, pitch level of the head etc.) according to the type of tone-group which precedes or follows it—should be considered in the analysis of normal connected discourse. Crystal discusses in some detail the sorts of predictable restrictions which operate on adjacent tone-groups; he finds, for example, a tendency towards repetition of the same tone pattern in sequence, particularly the pattern 'plus' where' represents a rising tone.

It is plausible that normal inter-tone-group relationships will be impaired in those disorders involving neuromuscular malfunctioning of the respiratory or the laryngeal systems. For example, the cricothyroid muscle, which is the main pitch-regulating muscular force in the larynx, may be affected by paralysis of the superior laryngeal nerve, or the respiratory muscles may be affected, so preventing the necessary air-flow through the glottis, which potentially influences not only the rate of vibration of the vocal cords (the fundamental frequency) but also the acoustic intensity of the resulting sound. In some of the dysarthrias, particularly that associated with Parkinsonism, a marked inability to produce the necessary pitch and intensity range for normal speech has been found. Darley, Aronson and Brown (1975) list the following as prominent characteristics of Parkinsonism: monotony of pitch, monotony of loudness, reduction of proper stress for emphasis, lower than average pitch level, inappropriate silences and excessively short phrases separated by pauses. All these features could potentially affect an assessment of overall speech fluency (see chapter 8).

Pausing

The frequency, distribution and duration of pauses have often been considered in assessments of speech fluency (see chapter 1). However, one of the difficulties in using aspects of pausing as indices of fluency arises from the fact that normal spontaneous speech is what Goldman-Eisler (1968, 31) calls 'a highly fragmented and discontinuous activity', and it is somewhat difficult to decide whether a particular pausing pattern is indicative of normal nonfluency or pathological disfluency. By discontinuous, Goldman-Eisler was referring primarily to the presence of gaps in the acoustic signal, those periods of silence which alternate with periods where speech sound is present. Three types of discontinuities or gaps are listed:

those associated with the articulatory closure of stop consonants
those occurring during an inhalatory phase when air is drawn into the lungs (so-called 'breath-pauses')
those seemingly unrelated to any articulatory processes (e.g. so-called 'hesitation' pauses)

Such discontinuities are obviously important in an assessment of fluency, and our main aim in this chapter will be to indicate some aspects of their distribution and function in normal speech and to suggest how the normal pattern can be altered in the pathological situation.

The first type of discontinuity is that associated with an articulatory stop closure and may range in duration from 50 msec. to as much as 250 msec., depending partly on such factors as the place of closure, the manner of closure, the articulatory organ or organs involved, the surrounding sounds, and suprasegmental features such as rhythm, stress or overall utterance rate. Often a sequence of two or more overlapping closures occur where the acoustic manifestation will still be a single period of silence. In the articulation of a word such as 'apt', for example, part of the alveolar closure for [t] will occur simultaneously with the lip closure for [p], which is normally unexploded in English. The period of silence associated with such a coarticulated sequence will normally be much longer than that caused by a single stop closure.

Discontinuities resulting from these stop closures are normally not considered pauses and become important in an assessment of fluency only when they are prolonged to such an extent that they are regarded by listeners as interrupting the flow of speech. In the first part of this chapter we saw how one of the frequent manifestations of certain pathological conditions, e.g. stuttering, may be a disfluent prolongation of stop closures, resulting for example from an abnormally high muscular tension in the articulatory organs involved. It was seen how this disfluent prolongation may contribute to a breakdown in the smooth coordination between the three speech physiological systems—the supraglottal (articulatory), laryngeal, and subglottal (respiratory) systems.

The second main type of discontinuity occurring in the speech signal is that associated with inhalation. These so-called 'breath pauses' occur at the end of

the exhalatory cycle when the speaker needs to replenish his air supply for biological reasons and in order to maintain a sufficiently high subglottal pressure for
the production of speech sounds. Most investigators have noted a close correlation
between the location of breath pauses and boundaries between syntactic units
such as clauses and sentences. Thus Sweet (1877, 42, 1890, 86–7):

> The only division actually made in language is that into 'breath groups'. These
> breath groups correspond partially to the logical division into sentences: every
> sentence is necessarily a breath group, but every breath group need not be a complete
> sentence. . . .

and Goldman-Eisler (1968, 99):

> During passages of prose read aloud, breaths were taken exclusively at gaps in
> speech designated as grammatical junctures. During spontaneous speech
> approximately one-third of the breaths were taken at gaps which could not be so
> described. . . .

A number of studies of breath pauses undertaken by Goldman-Eisler (see
summary in Goldman-Eisler 1968) showed that for normal speakers reading
English aloud these pauses range in average duration from 0·5 to 1 sec., and occur
at rates of between 2 and 20 per minute. For normal speakers the rate and duration
of such pauses is probably related to overall speed of utterance—the greater the
overall tempo the shorter and more frequent the pauses. Also for normal speakers,
the breath pauses are usually silent pauses, i.e. they are not accompanied by any
vocalization, although they may be heard as an audible voiceless hissing caused by
the generation of turbulent air at various points of stricture in the vocal tract. The
situation may be quite different with pathological speakers. Frequently patients
who lack precise control over the coordination between the articulatory, laryngeal
and respiratory systems, such as some dysarthric patients, particularly those with
Parkinson's disease and with bulbar palsy, may exhibit involuntary vocalization
during the inhalatory pause. (Darley, Aronson and Brown (1969) mention audible
inhalation as one of the characteristics of bulbar palsy and the dysarthria associated
with amyotrophic lateral sclerosis.) Such involuntary vocalization may occur, for
example, if the patients fail to abduct the vocal cords sufficiently to allow the ingressive air to pass relatively unimpeded through the glottis. An involuntary adduction
of the cords during an inhalatory flow of air may create conditions favourable for
voicing although, because of the ingressive air-stream direction, the mode of
vibration of the cords will be somewhat different from that characteristic of normal
egressive speech and an abnormal voice quality will be produced.

One can assume that the demands placed on the respiratory system during
normal speech are relatively slight (for typical subglottal pressures and flow rates
see Hixon 1966); it is normally sufficient simply to maintain the subglottal pressure
at a level suitably high to create the transglottal pressure conditions necessary
for voicing. For the pathological speaker, however, considerably greater demands

may be placed on the respiratory system. For example, if the supraglottal pressure level is generally higher than it is in normals, as some have suggested in the case with certain stutterers (see Adams 1974), the subglottal pressure required to produce speech may be correspondingly greater, as the difference between the supraglottal and subglottal pressures is still necessary for the appropriate transglottal air-flow and so vocalization (see chapter 7). For those stutterers and for some dysarthric groups, the aerodynamic energy expended by the respiratory system is probably greater than for normal speakers (see Hardy 1967). This increased energy may result in the need for more frequent replenishing of the air-supply than for normal speakers and thus more frequently occurring inhalations per unit time. The frequency of inhalations also may depend indirectly on the neuromuscular condition of muscles which control the tension and degree of adduction/abduction of the vocal cords. Should there be any reduction in the force and range of laryngeal muscular contraction, unwanted leakage of air may occur at the glottis. This could be associated with breathy voice quality and is characteristic of a number of pathological conditions such as unilateral paralysis of the vocal cords and some types of dysarthria. The leakage of air through the glottis could conceivably also contribute to the premature exhalation of the available air supply and result in the need for more frequent inhalations than for the normal speaker.

The frequency of breath pauses, then, may be a useful index of certain pathological conditions and may be related to various factors such as supra- and subglottal pressures, air-flow and the volume of air supply (vital capacity). Experiments (e.g. by Laszewski 1956) have already shown that patients with Parkinson's disease tend to have reduced vital capacities.

Not only the frequency of the breath pauses but their duration also can be affected in certain of the dysarthrias. Following damage to those lower motor neurones of the cranial nerves important for speech (particularly V, VII, IX, X and XII), patients may exhibit a general reduction in the force and range of muscular contraction often resulting in severe 'flaccidity' (Darley, Aronson and Brown 1975). One would expect in these cases a general undershooting of target articulations (see above under transition smoothness) and a general slowing down of all articulatory activity and corresponding respiratory functions. The speech of these patients, then, may conceivably be characterized by relatively long breath pauses, although at the present time very little experimental data exist to test that view.

Pauses which are not related directly to articulatory processes form the third main group in our classification of discontinuities. The location of these pauses, and the possible function they serve for both the speaker and listener, have received considerable attention from both linguists and psychologists—from the former because of their potential importance in signalling basic syntactic encoding units and from the latter because of their correlation with cognitive processes and affective states of the speaker.

Excellent reviews of the literature relating to the significance of these non-articulatory pauses are to be found in Rochester 1973 and Butcher 1973, 1975. We do not propose to replicate such reviews in this section, but simply to indicate the relevance of pausal phenomena in differentiating normal nonfluency from pathological disfluency. It will be necessary therefore to discuss on the one hand the main non-articulatory functions of pauses that have been proposed by various investigators and the conditions under which they occur, and on the other hand how the normal pausing pattern may change in pathological speech.

The occurrence of pauses in normal speech has been found to be associated with a number of non-articulatory variables including:

boundaries between syntactic and prosodic units such as the sentence, clause, phrase, tone group etc. (e.g. Lounsbury 1954, Boomer 1965, Johnson 1965, Martin, Roberts and Collins 1968, Henderson, Goldman-Eisler and Skarbeck 1966, Wilkes and Kennedy 1969, Hawkins 1971, Goldman-Eisler 1972, Ruder 1973)

cognitive functions influenced, for example, by lexical choices (e.g. Maclay and Osgood 1959, Goldman-Eisler 1958, Preston and Gardner 1967, Reynolds and Paivio 1968, Taylor 1969), and abstractness or difficulty of the task (e.g. Goldman-Eisler 1961a, Siegman and Pope 1965, 1966, Levin, Silverman and Ford 1967, Lay and Paivio 1969)

affective state of the speaker, for example situational anxiety (e.g. Mahl 1956, Kasl and Mahl 1965, Siegman and Pope 1965) and dispositional anxiety (e.g. Murray 1971)

social interaction variables (e.g. Maclay and Osgood 1959)

stylistic factors

In most of these studies a distinction is drawn between a silent or 'unfilled' pause (SP or UP), and a filled pause (FP) which contains a 'nonlexical intrusive sound' such as [ε], [aː], [m], [ʌm], [ə] etc. The relative locations of both types of pauses were noted by Maclay and Osgood (1959). In their analysis they found both sorts of pauses were more likely to occur before content words (e.g. nouns, verbs, adjectives) than before function words (e.g. prepositions, verbal auxiliaries etc.) although their relative distribution was slightly different. A filled pause was relatively more likely to occur before function words and at phrase boundaries (using the syntactic frames of Fries 1952), while silent pauses were more likely to occur before content words and within phrases. They suggested furthermore a specific function of filled pauses in signalling to the listener that the speaker wishes to keep control of the 'conversational ball'. Therefore if the speaker pauses long enough to receive the cue of his own silence he will produce some kind of signal [m, r] or perhaps a repetition of the immediately preceding unit) which says, in effect, 'I'm still in control—don't interrupt me!' (Maclay and Osgood 1959, 41). According to the authors, FPs tend to occur just before points of highest uncertainty and would most likely follow long silences. This latter hypothesis has since been challenged (e.g. by Boomer 1965, Lalljee and Cook 1969 and Goldman-Eisler 1961b).

The 'conversational ball' suggestion of Maclay and Osgood remains an attractive hypothesis and could be extended as proposed by Rochester (1973). He suggests that if long pauses typically result in a loss of control of the 'conversational ball' it follows that speakers should utter shorter pauses when they wish to maintain such control. Moreover, to the extent that any silence is an opportunity for a transfer of control, the speaker who wishes to continue speaking should utter fewer S.P.s (silent pauses) of all durations. There are several predictions which derive from this hypothesis. If the speaker's desire to maintain control of a conversation is signalled by an increase in F.P.s and a decrease in both duration and frequency of S.P.s then (1) these events should be more likely in dialogues than in monologues, (2) they should be less likely where the subject wishes to break off speaking, (3) they should be unchanged where the number of potential speakers remains constant, and (4) they should be more likely where the speaker lacks visual means of controlling the conversation. (75)

Rochester cites experimental evidence to support all four predictions.

The effects of cognitive functions and affective-state variables on the relative distribution of filled and unfilled pauses have been measured by a number of investigators with somewhat conflicting results. Two studies, Siegman and Pope 1965 and Reynolds and Paivio 1968 suggest that both FPs and UPs increase as a function of presumed difficulty of the experimental task. Goldman-Eisler (1961b) on the other hand, found that the frequency of FPs remained constant as the task difficulty increased (formulating the essential point of cartoon stories). Affective state altered by situational anxiety also seems to produce a differential effect on UPs and FPs. Most studies have found a positive correlation between situational anxiety and UPs, but not FPs (see Krause and Pilisuk 1961, Siegman and Pope 1965). These results are quite relevant to the present discussion particularly as regards stutterers, where one would expect a high level of situational anxiety epsecially in those communication situations where the stutterer feels most ill at ease (see chapter 7).

The present position as regards the relative distribution and function of filled and unfilled pauses seems, then, somewhat confused. We would tend to agree with Crystal's (1969, 169) assessment that 'the linguistic significance of the [FP/ UP] dichotomy has yet to be shown'.

The remainder of this section will be devoted to a more detailed discussion of the main variables affecting the distribution and function of pauses.

Syntactic correlates

The possible function of pauses in marking boundaries between syntactic units such as phrases, clauses and sentences has received considerable attention in the literature (see for example Lounsbury 1954, Boomer 1965, Barik 1968, Hawkins 1971, Goldman-Eisler 1972 and other references mentioned above). Many of these investigators have regarded the existence of pauses separating these syntactic units (so-called 'juncture pauses') as evidence for the reality of such units as neural encoding elements in the speech production process (see chapter 2).

One may speculate that the speaker makes a pause at the beginning of a syntactic unit such as a clause or phrase because it is at this point that his brain is pre-programming the following stretch of speech. Such a pause would then be viewed as a necessary result of a decision-making process and would be a predictable part of normal fluent speech (Boomer 1965). A pause, then, occurring at the boundaries between syntactic clauses would presumably aid intelligibility by imparting to the listener important syntactic cues. Such a pause would not be regarded as interrupting the flow of speech unless, of course, its duration was longer than one would normally expect at such locations. Abnormally long pauses may occur in the speech of some stutterers where the duration of the neural programming stage takes longer than normal, particularly if the stutterer is devising specific strategies to avoid difficult words etc. (see chapter 7).

Presumably, as far as the listener is concerned, the detection threshold of pauses in syntactic boundary positions would be higher than, for example, in an intra-phrase position because the listener's expectations would be biased in favour of a longer pause occurring at the syntactic boundaries. Such a result has been supported by experiments carried out by Boomer and Dittman (1962).

It is generally agreed, therefore, that pause duration is normally greater at the boundaries of syntactic units such as clauses than between individual words within a clause. There also seems to be a relationship between the incidence of pause and the type of clause involved. Goldman-Eisler (1972) examined pause duration in spontaneous speech and found that between words within clauses 93·1 per cent of transitions were 'fluent'—i.e. shorter than 0.5 sec., while relative subordinate clauses had 62·8 per cent fluent transitions, other subordinate clauses 50·7 per cent and coordinate clauses only 33·2 per cent.

Some investigators have suggested that the relative duration of pauses may conceivably reflect the complexity of the encoding process (see review in Rochester 1973). A measure of complexity would conceivably be the number of encoding processes which will be related to the syntactic structure of the sentence. For example, in a syntactic analysis of the sentence 'the girl who left you was here', the following diagram could be used to illustrate the hypothetical encoding operations that may take place:

1st encoding stage:	the girl who left you/was here
	Subject /Predicate
2nd encoding stage:	the girl/ who left you /was /here
	Subject /Predicate
	Noun phrase/modifying clause/verb/adverb
3rd encoding stage:	the girl/ who / left / you /was /here
	Subject /Predicate
	Noun phrase/ modifying clause /verb/adverb
	Noun phrase/pronoun/verb/pronoun/verb/adverb

One could hypothesize that a pause separating subject and predicate in the first stage would be longer than that in the third stage separating the relative pronoun from the verb, because of the relatively higher number of encoding operations remaining to be completed at the first stage. Such an index of syntactic complexity has been formulated by Miller and Chomsky (1963) and used by Ruder and Jensen (1972).

The structural function of pauses discussed so far presupposes a hierarchical process in the encoding of a sentence whereby structural syntactic decisions are made first followed by the lexical choices (selection of words). This is a very specific view of the encoding process of speech (cf. Chomsky 1965) which must remain speculative. One may just as easily hypothesize that lexical and syntactic decisions are made simultaneously (Rochester 1973). There is some suggestion in the literature (e.g. Taylor 1969) that pause duration and frequency have a functional relationship not with the syntactic encoding operation but with the 'content' of the sentence. The question however must remain open, as it is difficult to determine from the rather restricted laboratory conditions of experiments such as Taylor's the situation that obtains in natural spontaneous speech.

Cognitive variables

In a number of experiments Goldman-Eisler (see summaries in Goldman-Eisler 1968) suggested that pauses could reflect not only decisions at major syntactic boundaries but also decisions involving choices of words. According to this theory, after the speaker has uttered the first word of a sentence, only decisions involving selection of lexical items remain. Pauses may occur at such lexical selection points, the incidence of such pauses being related to the 'informational content' of the following word and its 'transitional probability'. An experiment using a modification of the Shannon guessing technique (Goldman-Eisler 1958) showed that words following intra-phrase pauses were less predictable (i.e. had a lower transitional probability) than words in a fluent context. A distinction is drawn between utterances which consist of well-established, habitual sequences such as clichés or greetings and less habitual, more creative sequences such as the expression of abstract concepts. Utterances of the former type supposedly have more temporal cohesion and therefore contain relatively fewer and shorter pauses than utterances of the latter type. Goldman-Eisler suggested furthermore that, for normal speakers, relatively long periods of fluency alternate with periods of hesitancy in a relatively long-term cyclic fashion (Goldman-Eisler 1968, 94; see also Henderson, Goldman-Eisler and Skarbeck 1965, 1966). Presumably, during the periods of hesitancy, creative planning for the following utterances is being carried out.

The correlation between the incidence of pauses and lexical choices has been supported by Preston and Gardner (1967) who found persons with poor vocabularies paused more frequently and for longer periods than those with good vocabularies. The pause time is evidently taken up by the speaker searching his lexical store for the right word (see chapter 2). Some pathological speakers, particularly those aphasics with difficulty in word selection, will invariably pause longer and more frequently than normal speakers. The word-selection disorder has been described in detail by Luria (1973) and Goldstein (1948) and is said to arise most frequently from damage to the parieto-occipital zone of the dominant cerebral hemisphere. The patients have particular difficulty in naming objects and will often use a variety of substitutes for the correct word. These substitute words are frequently related in some way to the required word either semantically, phonetically or grammatically, and the situation facing these aphasics is probably analogous to a normal speaker's attempts to recall a momentarily forgotten name or object.

Another cognitive variable potentially affecting the frequency and location of pauses is the situational task difficulty. Attempts to vary task difficulty under laboratory conditions, e.g. by getting subjects to define abstract rather than concrete nouns (Reynolds and Paivio 1968) or discussing TAT cards (i.e. Thematic Apperception Test cards, which depict some real-life situation) increasing in ambiguity (Siegman and Pope 1966) have shown that, in general, both filled and unfilled pauses increase as a function of the increase in the presumed task difficulty. An analogous situation can be found among pathologically disfluent speakers such as stutterers, whose stuttering manifestations increase with task difficulty.

Affective-state correlates

Most work carried out exploring the relationship between the frequency and duration of pauses and variables concerning the affective state of the speaker, such as increased situational or predispositional anxiety, has been done by psychologists (e.g. Mahl 1956, Krause and Pilisuk 1961, Siegman and Pope 1965, Murray 1971). The general consensus seems to be that UPs increase in duration and frequency as situational anxiety is heightened. The results for FPs seem somewhat less conclusive. In the light of these findings it may be important in the rehabilitation of patients with various types of pathological disfluencies (especially stutterers) to note those situations in everyday communication which the patient finds particularly stressful. One would expect (and we shall find in chapter 7) that the speech of such patients in these situations may be characterized by increased duration and frequency of pauses, so compounding their already existing disfluency problem.

Social-interaction variables

In typical face-to-face communication there is a great deal of subtle interaction between the speaker and the listener. The speaker, for example, is usually extremely aware of the response of the listener to what he is saying and may use a wide variety of cues, both linguistic and paralinguistic, to keep the listener's interest, invite him actively to participate in the interchange etc. Some of the possible functions of FPs in the communication situation have already been mentioned above with reference to the 'conversational ball' hypothesis of Maclay and Osgood (1959). If, as suggested by Rochester (1973), Maclay and Osgood's hypothesis is extended to include UPs, then long pauses would result in a loss of control of the 'conversational ball' and speakers should use relatively shorter pauses if they wished to maintain such control. To date attempts to test the Maclay and Osgood hypothesis (e.g. by Lalljee and Cook (1969)) have been somewhat inconclusive mainly because of the extreme artificiality of the experimental situation (see Rochester 1973).

Stylistic variables

The use of pauses both filled and unfilled for stylistic reasons is well known amongst professional speakers such as newscasters and politicians. As a rhetorical device pauses are often used by such people to add emphasis to a particular word or to impart some special emotive colouring. For example in the sequence 'it must have been a // frightful sight', a pause would not normally occur between 'a' and 'frightful' unless the speaker wanted to place particular emphasis on the word 'frightful'. In such cases the intonation pattern also may be modified to contribute to the added emphasis, e.g. a high fall nuclear tone occurring on the first syllable of 'frightful'.

Another rhetorical device frequently employed by broadcasters is the use of a pause as a finality marker (see Abercrombie 1968) to signal, for example, that the speaker is coming to the end of what he has to say. This may occur in the last item of a news broadcast, for example 'the inquiry into the accident // opens tomorrow'. Abercrombie (1968) regards this type of pause as a 'silent stress', which he defines as a place where a stress would normally occur due to the rhythmical pattern of the language, but does not. He claims that, with reference to examples like the above, the more silent stresses there are the greater will be the degree of finality, e.g. 'you'll hear all about it // at ten fifty // in // Grandstand'.

Unexpected or unusual placement of pauses is another frequent stylistic device used by professional broadcasters. Abercrombie gives an example of this idio-syncratic use of pausing: 'He has to be all things to // all men', where the pause (Abercrombie's 'silent stress') after 'to' appears to serve no useful purpose other than to contribute to variation in the basic rhythmical pattern. Further examples may be found in Crystal and Davy (1969).

Rhythmical patterning

Another index of speech fluency is rhythmical patterning, which refers here to a temporal sequencing of similar events. The 'similar events' may be those syllables which 'stand out' or are more prominent than their neighbours, the prominence being signalled to the listener by a variety of acoustic cues such as increased duration of vowel nuclei, change in pitch, and increased intensity. The occurrence of these so-called rhythmical stresses in English can be illustrated by the following passage spoken with a normal intonation pattern:

'/Can't he ac/count for the /two /cases/?'

The strokes / indicate boundaries between rhythmical units, and each of these rhythmical units has a stress on the first syllable (i.e. on 'can't', '-count', 'two' and 'cas-'). There appears to be a tendency in English for these rhythmical stresses to occur at roughly equal intervals of time and this general *isochronicity* is said to characterize the rhythmical structure of English (see Abercrombie 1965). The tendency towards isochronicity means that the duration of syllables in each rhythmical unit is adjusted according to the number of syllables in that unit. In the above example, the duration of the two syllables in 'cases' (comprising the last rhythmical unit) would be roughly equal to the combined duration of the three syllables in '-count', 'for' and 'the' (comprising the second rhythmical unit). What happens normally is that the unstressed vowels in the rhythmical unit (e.g. those in 'for' and 'the') are reduced in duration and assume a quality approaching that of the centralized unstressed vowel [ə] as occurs initially in the word 'above'. It should be emphasized here that isochronicity in English rhythmical stresses is seen as a general *tendency* only—measurement of the precise duration between successive stressed syllables reveals considerable variability, particularly in connected speech (Allen 1972, 1975).

Most rhythmical units (or 'metric feet' as they are sometimes called) in English comprise two or three syllables, and there is a tendency normally to avoid juxta-position of two stresses. Thus in two sequences '/come to the /upstairs /bedroom /' and '/Bob /went up-/stairs' the stress in 'upstairs' shifts according to the rhythmical stress environment—in the first example the syllable preceding 'upstairs' is unstressed and in the second example it is stressed; so in order to avoid a juxta-position of two stresses, the stress in the second example is shifted to the second syllable in 'upstairs' (see Allen 1975).

The rate of succession of rhythmical units in English for normal speakers in conversational utterances has been measured at between 0·3 and 0·6 sec. (Allen 1972). Allen (1975) sees a parallel between this rate and that of motor acts in general. He cites research by Miyake (1902) and Woodrow (1951) which shows that all motor activity is rhythmical and the 'preferred' rates for motor acts are two per second (i.e. one every 0·5 sec.). As speech articulation is a type of motor activity, it is not surprising to find the rate of rhythmical 'beats' or stresses in speech corresponding to that of bodily activity.

Languages differ in the rhythmical patterning of their speech utterances. English rhythm, as we have shown, is characterized by a roughly isochronous succession of rhythmical stressed syllables, and a 'reduction' of intervening unstressed syllables, the degree of reduction being proportional to the number of such syllables. A less marked tendency for reduction of unstressed syllables, however, is shown in languages such as Spanish and French. In these languages the duration of unstressed syllables is rarely reduced to the same extent as in English, nor is the phonetic quality of the syllabic vowel nucleus so altered. The rhythmical structure of these languages appears to be based more on a succession of syllables than on rhythmical stresses. For this reason some linguists (e.g. Pike 1945) have referred to English as a 'stress-timed' language and to French and Spanish as 'syllable-timed' languages. Although it is difficult to imagine a neat division of all the languages of the world into either 'syllable-timed' or 'stress-timed' (cf. Mitchell's (1969) review of Abercrombie), nevertheless, the terms may be usefully employed as broad general labels in the description of rhythmical structure in a particular language.

Breakdown in normal rhythmical patterning is seen as a characteristic of a number of pathological conditions including many of the dysarthrias, particularly that associated with Parkinsonism and ataxic dysarthria (see Darley, Aronson and

Brown 1975). The term 'scanning speech' has been applied to a type of disrhythmia, one of the main features of which has been described by Darley, Aronson and Brown (1975) as: 'a seeming equalization of stress on words and syllables that do not warrant equal stress and the use of excess stress on words and syllables that do not appear to warrant it'. They call this feature 'excess and equal stress' and regard it in their analysis of the dysarthrias as the second most prominent feature of dysarthria resulting from disease of the cerebellum with the associated prosodic features 'prolongation of phonemes', 'prolongations of intervals between phonemes' and 'slow rate' (Darley, Aronson and Brown 1975, 167). The rhythmic feature of 'excess and equal stress' is reminiscent of a sort of exaggerated syllable-timed rhythmical pattern, the main features of which we discussed above. It is also interesting to note that one technique frequently used to improve disfluency is the use of syllable-timed speech (see chapter 7).

Regulation of tempo

The fourth potential feature which we consider primarily important in an assessment of speech fluency is regulation of overall tempo or rate of utterance. For normal speakers tempo is adjusted according to such factors as stylistic effects, biological demands on the speech system, cognitive processing, and will normally be limited by the physiological systems—such factors as the intrinsic speed of articulatory activity and the transmission time for motor impulses to the speech muscles being primarily important. The overall rate will be affected also by the duration and frequency of pauses; in fact it has been suggested that the overall rate of speech production is reflected mainly in terms of time taken up by hesitation pauses (Goldman-Eisler 1968, 31).

There are a number of ways of measuring overall utterance rate, one of the most useful being the number of syllables articulated each second in a stretch of speech. This number has been found to be about 6 ± 1 for normal speakers (see Lenneberg 1967). This rate of syllable production must obviously be limited to some extent by the speed of individual articulatory movements, which, according to measurements carried out by Hudgins and Stetson (1937) range from 5·2 to 9·6 per second, with the tongue tip being capable of the fastest speed. The syllable rate of 6 ± 1 falls roughly midway within this range.

Clearly the overall utterance rate will be affected when articulatory movement is slowed down, for example, in most of the dysarthrias. We have already seen earlier in this chapter how some pathological conditions can affect the coordination between speech physiological systems and result in a breakdown of smooth transitions between adjacent speech sounds and syllables. Such uncoordination will usually result in a slower rate of utterance than normal. Pausing also will affect the overall rate, and we saw earlier how the frequency, duration and location of pauses can be influenced both by physiological conditions (such as respiratory requirements) and also by cognitive variables.

In certain pathological conditions such as cluttering and some forms of Parkinsonism (see chapter 8), there is an increased rate of utterance rather than a slowing down, and this has certain predictable effects on speech articulation. In the case of cluttering, which may involve a breakdown in the neural control mechanism responsible for temporal ordering (see chapter 2), the increased rate of utterance results in a greater degree of coarticulation than normal, and frequently also the elision of sounds or even whole syllables. We have seen earlier in this chapter an instance of normal coarticulation in the lip-rounding of the initial stop consonant in the word 'too'. Such coarticulation normally operates regressively or from right to left in English and can affect both place and manner of articulation (see Gimson 1970, Daniloff and Hammarberg 1973, Ladefoged 1975). Further examples of typical right-to-left coarticulation of place in normal speech are the following :

'key' — [kiː] with [k] having a pre-velar place of articulation because of the following close front vowel

'core' — [kɔː] with [k] having a post-velar place of articulation because of the following half-open back vowel

'width' — [wɪdθ] with [d] having a dental place of articulation under the influence of the following inter-dental fricative [θ]

'I'm' — [aɪm] with slight nasalization on the [ɪ] due to the lowering of the soft palate for the following [m]

The extent of coarticulatory influence in the above examples appears limited to one sound segment only (the preceding one). However, investigations have shown that coarticulatory processes can extend over two or even three sounds (Amerman, Daniloff and Moll 1970, Moll and Daniloff 1971) and can operate in both directions (i.e. left to right as well as right to left). There is some evidence also that coarticulation is influenced by syntactic considerations such as word and syllable boundaries (Kozhevnikov and Chistovich 1965). It is plausible that the speech of clutterers may be characterized by a greater degree of coarticulation than is normal, with coarticulatory influence extending over more than four segments, for example, and not being constrained by word and syllable boundaries.

The coarticulatory processes we have discussed so far result in allophonic variations and are normally obligatory, i.e. beyond the conscious control of the speaker. Other similar processes, however, involve phonemic variations and are mostly optional. Examples are:

'that pen' — /ˈðæp ˌpen/

'this ship' — /ˈðɪʃ ˌʃɪp/

'ten men' — /ˈtem ˌmen/

'good morning' — /ˌgʊm ˈmɔːnɪŋ/

It can be seen that most of these coarticulatory processes involve alveolars, and the tendency of alveolar consonants to assimilate in place of articulation has been noted in the literature (e.g. Gimson 1970).

All of these coarticulations are more marked under conditions of increased overall utterance rate.

Another phonetic effect of increased overall utterance rate in normal speech is the tendency towards omission or elision of speech sounds. In the normal speaker this is confined largely to the omission of single segments only; however, more than one consonant segment may be elided in some three- or four-term consonant clusters. Typical sound omissions in fast colloquial speech are as follows (examples mostly from Gimson, 1970):

Omission of vowels:	'not alone'—/'nɒtl̩ 'ləʊn/ (omission of /ə/ in /ələʊn/)
	'father and son'—/'fɑːðrən ˌsʌn/ (omission of /ə/ in /fɑːðə/)
Omission of consonants:	'next day'—/'neks 'deɪ/ (omission of /t/ in /nekst/)
	'already'—/ˌɔːˈredɪ/ (omission of /l/)
	'lastly'—/'lɑːsliː/ (omission of /t/)

An analysis of the main examples of consonant elisions shows that most involve the alveolar place of articulation.

Many of the phonetic features of the pathological disorder of cluttering are similar to those manifested in normal fast colloquial speech, particularly the coarticulations, elisions and reduction in duration and quality of the so-called weak forms of vowels. However, frequently in cluttered speech whole syllables and words are omitted, rather than single segments as is usual in normal speech. The omission of these larger units, together with the greater degree of coarticulation, often contributes to a severe reduction in intelligibility. Also in cluttering, the overall utterance rate may be so fast that there is not enough time for adequate pre-programming of the speech utterances, so that syntactic structures in the speech output appear somewhat jumbled and inappropriate for the idea being expressed.

So far in this section we have discussed some of the main phonetic manifestations of both reduced overall speed of utterance and increased overall speed. For the normal speaker there is relatively little variability of tempo in a given communication situation; any changes that occur in the rate result mainly from different affective-state, stylistic or cognitive requirements. For some dysarthric speakers, however, particularly Parkinson patients, regulation of tempo, i.e. the ability to maintain a relatively constant rate of utterance, poses a severe problem. Speech in these patients is frequently characterized by 'sudden rushes' (Darley, Aronson and Brown 1975), as if the patient were trying to complete a syntactic unit the size of a tone-group as quickly as possible before taking a breath.

This chapter has outlined some of the characteristics of the main indices that can be used in the assessment of speech fluency—transition smoothness including pausing patterns, rhythmical patterning, and regulation of tempo, as applied to both normal and pathological speech. In discussing the features of transition smoothness separately, however, we do not want to suggest that they are discrete independent variables. In fact as we pointed out in the last section on regulation of tempo, each of the indices can exert an influence on the others. This is not altogether surprising, as all are concerned with the temporal ordering of speech production.

The main variables affecting transition smoothness are summarized in the facing table. Following this table, Figs. 4 and 5 illustrate some of the main phonetic characteristics of the two disorders normally referred to as disorders of fluency—namely cluttering and stuttering.

In order to illustrate how some of these variables may be altered in pathological disfluency, the following diagrams are presented showing the main *phonetic* features which are potentially characteristic of the disorders of stuttering and cluttering as compared with normal nonfluencies. (Most of these features are exemplified in the transcription of stuttered speech in the appendix (p. 137)). It should be stressed that any two stutterers or clutterers will almost certainly differ in the way in which these features are manifested. Also the main distinguishing features of the disorder may lie elsewhere than in the overt phonetic manifestations: for example, in the use of circumlocution in word avoidances, in facial gestures accompanying a hard block etc. Such features will de discussed more fully in chapter 7. In the following chapters attention will be focused mainly on the disorders of stuttering and cluttering which are classified as disorders of fluency, i.e. those disorders which manifest pathological disfluencies in the absence of the sorts of neuromuscular impairments one finds in the dysarthrias.

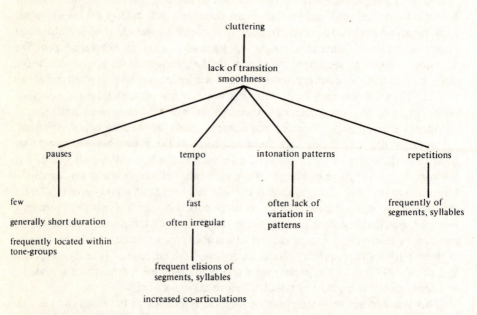

Fig. 4.   Diagram showing some of the typical manifestations of cluttering

transition smooth-ness				
	prosodic level	pauses	physiological (breath pauses)	filled unfilled
			nonphysiological	filled unfilled
		tempo	fast	increased elisions increased coarticulations
			slow irregular	
		intonation patterns	interactions between adjacent tone groups variability in intonation patterns	
		rhythmical patterns	mainly 'stress-timed' mainly 'syllable-timed'	
	segmental phonetic level	prolongations (of segments)	articulated with increased muscular tension articulated normally	affects the co-ordination between supraglottal, laryngeal and sub-glottal systems
		tension in speech muscles	abnormally high muscular tension abnormally low muscular tension	
		blocks ('hard attacks' 'hard contacts')	tensely-articulated stop closures	
			glottal-stop initiations of vowels	
		repetitions	of sounds of syllables	
	grammatical level	syntactic 'links'	use of coordinators use of subordinators	
			repetitions	of words of phrases of clauses
		morphological 'links'	use of inflexional endings	
		linking of thematic elements	incomplete phrases revisions	
	lexical/ semantic level	use of lexical items		
		miscellaneous discontinuities	interjections interruptions	

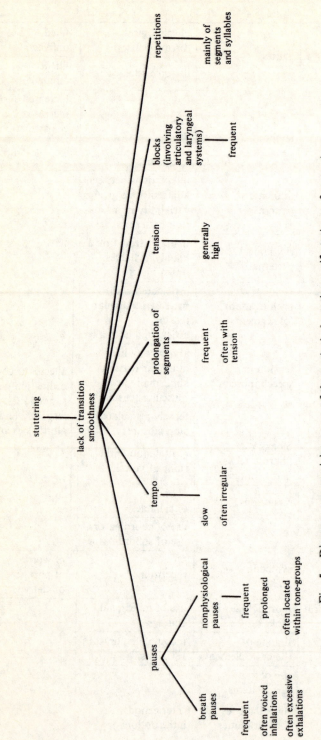

Fig. 5. Diagram summarizing some of the typical phonetic manifestations of stuttering

4

Developments in linguistic profiling of stuttering

Quantitative measures of stuttering

In the previous chapter we outlined some of the motoric and linguistic factors which could usefully be taken into account in an assessment of stuttering behaviour. In this chapter we aim to build on this theoretical background in proposing a framework for a profiling scheme which may be used to characterize a particular speaker's disability. In common with other profiling schemes of speech disorders (e.g. Crystal 1982) it seeks to provide the therapist with detailed relevant descriptive data on the speech of a particular individual for use in designing remedial programmes, and serve also as a useful framework on which to chart progress during a course of therapy.

A number of factors need to be taken into account in the design of an appropriate profile. Firstly the measures used need to be clinically relevant in that they should include those which have been mentioned previously in the literature as being potentially important for the characterization of pathological disfluency as distinct from normal non-fluency, although of course, as was pointed out in the previous chapters, this distinction is frequently far from clear-cut. A second requirement is that the profile should be relatively easy to compile and does not involve an inordinate amount of time on the part of therapist or client.

An important initial consideration in any assessment procedure is to decide on the type of speech sample to be used. Ideally, different types of speech material should be used, as it has been shown that fluency may be affected by a variety of factors, such as the subject matter of the sample, the recording environment, the nature of the audience etc. (see Costello and Ingham 1985). Costello and Ingham (1985) suggest for the assessment of children, speech samples should be obtained both within and outside the clinic. Within the clinic they suggest one 10 min. conversation between child and parent and one 10 min. conversation between child and clinician. Outside the clinic they suggest 10 min. stretches in at least 4 samples: (1) with the clinician outside the clinic room (2) at home with the other parent or similar guardian (3) at home with a sibling or frequent playmate (4) in a regularly occurring activity in the preschool or regular school setting. For adults they suggest samples also to be taken inside and outside the clinic; outside the clinic, 5 min. samples including: (1) conversation with the clinician (2) conversation with a spouse or close friend (3) telephone conversation with a friend (4) conversation occurring with someone in the workplace. Inside the clinic samples might include 5 mins. of oral reading, conversation between client and clinician and a monologue with the clinician absent. The rationale for using different types of sample is that stutterers may manifest quite different disfluent symptoms in the different speech situations. For example a speaker may appear quite fluent in a normal conversation but will in fact be using word avoidance strategies. For this speaker, the reading task may in fact produce many more disfluency features than his normal conversation, because in reading he is unable to use his avoidance strategies. On the other hand, another speaker may find the monologue task far more difficult than reading, as he is forced here to initiate propositional speech. Conversation with the clinician may be more problematic still, as not only must he initiate speech, but he also has to observe the principles of communication interaction. It would obviously be desirable also to elicit the different speech samples on a variety of occasions, as stutterers may be quite variable in their responses to the same task from one day to the next.

Another problem for the assessment is the definition of what constitutes stuttering as distinct from normal non-fluency (see previous chapters). Wingate's (1964b) definition seems to be the most enduring: stuttering includes involuntary, audible and silent repetitions or prolongations in the utterance of short speech elements namely, sounds, syllables and words of one syllable. There are of course other overt and covert symptoms of so-called assessory features (see review in Andrews et al 1983; Van Riper 1982) which may or may not be present in any given stutterer, but Wingate's features seem to capture the essential characteristics of pathologically stuttered speech. They at least serve as a convenient basis for assessment purposes (for fuller discussion of problems of definition and similar issues see Curlee 1984; Perkins 1983).

A variety of motoric and linguistic features may be used in the assessment or profiling scheme. Costello and Ingham (1985) propose a number of global quantitative measures which include frequency of stuttering, duration of moments of stutterng, speed of speech and articulatory rate, length of stutter-free utterances and speech quality. For these measures no attempt is made to specify the exact phonetic characteristics of each incidence of stuttering: they are based on "moments of stuttering and one moment of stuttering is counted for each of the speaker's attempts to produce a given syllable, irrespective of the duration of that attempt" (Costello and Ingham 1983: 311). Frequency of stuttering is measured as the percentage of syllables stuttered in the speech sample. Duration of moments of stuttering captures some information on severity and is measured as the length in seconds of the client's typical moments of stuttering. An additional measure is the actual length of the three longest moments of stuttering for each speech sample. Overall speaking rate or speed of speech is measured in syllables spoken per minute (adult norm 190–210, Ingham 1984) although, as Costello and Ingham point out, this measure is not an accurate representation of the actual speed of speech because of pauses, long periods of disfluency etc. They suggest an additional measure of articulatory rate expressed as the syllable per minute measure on samples with no stutterings or other disfluencies, and from which pauses more than 2 sec. have been eliminated. Length of stutter-free utterances is measured in either seconds or syllables, a subsidiary measure being the length of the three longest stutter-free utterances. Speech quality is based on work by Martin et al (1984) where listeners rate speech "naturalness" on a 9 point scale (1=highly natural 9=highly unnatural). Ingham and Costello's (1985) measures give global indication only of each speaker's stuttering patterns and, because they rely on total counts, do not relate the particular incidences of disfluency to motoric and linguistic factors. But the location of each stuttering instance in relation to these factors may provide important indicators for characterizing the disorder in a particular individual, thus giving more precise indication of severity and also may be used in planning a specific therapy programme for that individual. We hypothesize that the location of a disfluency is not entirely random but will be subject to certain definable motoric, linguistic and psychological constraints. It should be possible to predict for any given speaker that a disfluency is more likely than not to occur at a particular location in the utterance, where a particular constellation of physiological, aerodynamic, linguistic, prosodic features co-occur.

As far as linguistic constraints are concerned, there is a long tradition correlating phonological, morphological and syntactic factors with stuttering behaviour. Early work by Brown (e.g. Brown 1937; 1945) established that stuttering in adults was more likely to occur on certain word classes (specifically adjectives, nouns, adverbs, mainly the so-called "content" words) than on others (e.g. prepositions, pronouns, conjunctions, articles, verbs, mainly so-called "function" words), was more likely in the early part of the sentence, more likely on long words beginning with a consonant than with a vowel, and on stressed rather than unstressed syllables. By and large these main tendencies have been substantiated in later studies (see reviews in St Louis, 1979; Bloodstein, 1981; Andrews et al, 1983) and some additional ones have been proposed including word frequency (e.g. Ronson 1976), "information loading" of words (e.g. Soderberg 1971), syllable position (MacKay and Soderberg 1970; quoted by Hamre, 1985), grammatical "complexity" e.g. length of sentence (Tornick and Bloodstein 1976) and various other semantic and pragmatic factors such as "propositionality" etc.

Of course, as St Louis (1979) clearly illustrates, there is considerable overlap between these different parameters, "content" words in general tend to be longer, less frequent, have greater information loading than "function" words and will also be more likely to carry the main linguistic stress. In fact, as Wingate (1985) points out, grammatical class and position in the sentence or clause may be simply an artifactual reflection of linguistic stress. Stress may in fact be the primary factor underlying many of the linguistic correlates that have been proposed in the past.

One of the problems with a traditional "parts of speech" approach such as the early work of Brown's is that the linguistic analysis is probably too simplistic in not taking into account the type of constituent structure in which the word occurs. The grammatical context in which the stuttered word occurs in fact may be more important than the word class itself. It has frequently been pointed out, for example, that the tendency for content words to be more closely associated with stuttering than function words may be confounded by the position and function in the syntactic structure or the type of structure. Soderberg (1967), for example, found that the unusually high percentage of stuttering on function words in his data appeared to reflect the fact that such words occurred most frequently in clause initial position. Hannah and Gardner (1968) also stressed the importance of the type of syntactic structure in the analysis of stuttering location. They carried out a syntactic analysis of their speech samples by segmenting the clauses into pre-verbal, verbal and post-verbal elements and found that stutterings which occurred in post-verbal elements of clauses varied as a function of how the post-verbal element was expanded (e.g. by phrase, clause, etc.). The prevalence of disfluency features associated with function words occurring at the beginnings of syntactic units has been noted for pre-school children (Helmreich and Bloodstein 1973; Silverman 1973) but, according to Gregory (1986), there is a transition to more stuttering or non-fluency features on content words as the children become older (4–8 years).

One of the general conclusions from the literature is that stuttering is more likely to occur at those locations in the stream of speech where major cognitive functions are being performed e.g. before relatively complex syntactic structures. There are clear parallels in this regard with the location of pauses (see chapter 3).

In the profiling scheme we should therefore specify not just the grammatical word class associated with the stuttering instance but its role as a constituent element in syntactic structure. In the profiling scheme proposed here based on that in Edwards and Hardcastle (1987) each word on which a particular disfluency occurs is identified as a constituent in either a phrase or clause and is logged in terms of its function: at the phrase level in terms of grammatical word-class (preposition, determiner, noun etc.) and at the clause level as occurring as the subject, verb, object, complement or adverbial element. (The categories used in this syntactic analysis are based on those proposed in the grammar of Quirk, Greenbaum, Leech, Svartvich (1972) and are widely known and used in speech therapy (see e.g. the linguistic profiling scheme LARSP, Crystal, Fletcher and Garman 1976)).

In addition to syntactic features such as those indicated above, the profiling scheme includes phonetic, (segmental) phonological and prosodic features associated with each moment of disfluency. One advantage of this approach is that by scoring each instance of disfluency in relation to its location at different levels we are able to predict whether, for a given speaker, a particular combination of phonetic, phonological, prosodic and syntactic variables is more likely to predispose stuttering behaviour than another.

Linguistic profiling procedure

The first stage in the profiling procedure is to obtain appropriate samples of speech. As mentioned above, it is desirable to obtain a variety of speech samples, if possible on a number of different occasions. Bearing in mind the practical limitations of the clinician's time and the relatively detailed nature of this profile it would not seem feasible to incorporate all Costello and Ingham's (1985) sample types (see above). We have compromised in suggesting a minimum of three different samples — a set passage to read; a monologue e.g. a picture description and a stretch of conversational speech (e.g. interview with the clinician). Separate profiles are completed for the first 100 words of each speech sample.

Each sample is video taped and an orthographic transcription made from the tape, marking tone units and each instance of a disfluency. Following Wingate (1964), the two core types of disfluency identified as manifestations of the lack of transition smoothness (see chapter 3 above), are repetitions (silent or audible) and prolongations (silent or audible). Repetitions may be elemental (i.e. segment or a consonant-vowel syllable where the vowel is of indeterminate central quality, schwa), phoneme cluster, syllable, word, phrase or clause. The rationale for regarding the C ə syllable as an elemental repetition and one of the characteristic features of stuttering is based on Van Riper's (1982) assertion that stutterers usually repeat not the target vowel but schwa (thus [bə bə bə bu:t] is more likely than [bu bu bu bu bu:t]). To count as an elemental repetition there should be a well defined reduplication of the element involved, and the reduplicated item should be similar in duration to the target segment. Prolongations, either audible or silent, involve an abnormal increase in the duration of a particular stage of phoneme production. For oral stop consonants and affricates, prolongation involves the closure phase and may or may not be accompanied by vocal fold vibration. For fricatives it involves prolongation of the stricture phase. Prolongations may be accompanied by intermittent voicing or periodic oscillations of the vocal organs. In fact it is quite likely that some abnormal laryngeal or respiratory activity may accompany the disfluency. (For a fuller discussion of laryngeal involvement in stuttering see Adams, Freeman and Conture 1985). No attempt is made in this profile to describe the precise phonetic character of such features. They are simply coded as prolongations with or without vocal oscillations (+ OSC in the profile chart) rather than as repetitions. Disfluencies are therefore logged under the target sound regardless of the precise phonetic nature of the disfluent element. For example, an abnormal mode of vibration of the vocal folds may accompany a prolonged /m/ in the word "money" (see sample text in Appendix A), or a prolongation may be accompanied by abnormal audible inhalation or aspiration as in [ʰr ə ʊ dz] (see Appendix A). In both cases the disfluent feature is scored as a prolongation on the initial consonant sounds /m/ and /r/.

Separate sections of the full profile are compiled for each of the two main disfluency features; repetitions and prolongations (Figs. 6 and 7). In addition, a profile of pausing patterns may be compiled (fig. 8), as the location, frequency and duration of pauses have been shown to be potentially relevant in a characterization of disorders of fluency (see chapter 3). The pauses identified for the purpose of this profile are those which cannot be easily accounted for in terms of articulatory activity. The prolonged closure phase of a stop, for example in the word "accountant" (see Excerpt 1 in the Appendix), would not score as a pause although detected as a clearly defined gap in the acoustic signal. It would be counted as a silent prolongation. "Breath" pauses, however, i.e. those accompanied by an inhalation, and "filled" pauses would however count as pauses for the purpose of the profile and would be scored according to location as are the prolongations and repetitions.

The actual profile charts for each of the three main sections; repetitions, prolongations and pauses are slightly different so will be discussed in turn.

Repetitions

The first 100 words of each speech sample is used as a basis for the profile. Repetitions that occur are divided into 6 subtypes; elemental, cluster, syllable, word, phrase or clause (see Fig. 6). The elemental repetitions involve a single phoneme, part of a phoneme or consonant phoneme plus schwa-type vowel. Each repetition is coded in terms of its frequency i.e. whether the element, cluster, syllable, word, phrase or clause is repeated once, twice, thrice, four or more times. The rationale for including repetition frequency in the profile is the oft-cited evidence in the literature that one of the ways in which a pathological stutter may be differentiated from a normal non-fluency is in the number of reduplications per stuttering instance (stuttering children average about two reiterations per instance according to Yaire and Lewis, 1984). The total length of each repetition instance (see Costello and Ingham 1985) and also the regularity of the rhythm or tempo during the repetition (Gregory and Hill 1984) may be additional relevant measures. In this profile we differentiate those repetitions which are slow by circling the appropriate repetition code. Frequently the slow repetitions are accompanied by increased muscular tension and it is such increases in tension that are said to be often relevant for differentiating stuttering from normal non-fluency (see e.g. Starkweather, Armson and Amster 1987).

The measures relating to number of reiterations per repetition instance and the rate of repetition instance allow, in this profile, a more refined representation of severity of stuttering than accounts which simply count the incidents of repetitions per 100 words. Assessments such as the latter would not distinguish between two stutterers both of whom have the same percentage of repetitions but differ in the severity of the repetition. The location of each repetition is considered where appropriate at four levels of analysis: prosodic, lexical, phrasal, clausal.

Prosodic level

As was seen in chapter 2 there is some indication in the literature that a prosodic unit such as the tone unit may be an important programming unit in the neural control of speech production. We therefore suggest its possible relationship to the location of instances of stuttering.

Following O'Connor and Arnold (1973) we identify three main parts of the one unit, the nucleus (carrying the main prominence and pitch movement of the unit) the head, that part of the tone unit before the nucleus, and the tail, that part after the nucleus. Some syllables in the head or tail may be more prominent than their neighbours by carrying a rhythmical stress (see chapter 3). Each repetition is located within the tone unit and the presence or absence of rhythmical stress associated with the tone unit noted also. The tail of the tone unit is normally relatively short in English and contains relatively few stressed syllables.

Lexical level

The location of elemental and cluster disfluencies in relation to the structure of the word is considered as either word initial or within the word. "Within word" is further subdivided into syllable initial or other. There are strong indications in the literature that most disfluencies occur syllable initially (e.g. Johnson and Brown 1935). The grammatical word class associated with the disfluency is specified under the phrase levels. The main classes used in this profile are adverbial (A), adjectival (Adj) auxiliary verb (Aux), coordinator (c), copular (cop), determiner (D), intensifier (Int), noun (N), negator (Neg), particle (part), preposition (Pr), pronoun (Pron) and subordinator (s).

Phrasal level

The phrase structure in which the disfluency occurs is logged under this section and the elements in the phrase listed. The word containing the disfluency is underlined. If the phrase itself has been repeated then the whole phrase is underlined.

Clausal level

Under the clausal level in the profile, each disfluency is located in the appropriate constituent by underlining. Five constituent elements in the clause are identified in this profile: Subject (S), Verb (V), Object (O), Complement (C) and Adverbial (A). When a constituent is expanded at either the phrase or clause level this is indicated by a stroke after the appropriate constituent element (e.g. O'). Occasionally a disfluency affects more than one element of the clause. For example in a two-word repetition, the first word may be part of the verbal element of the clause and the second word part of the object element. In such cases, when logging such a disfluency at the clause level, the two clausal elements involved in the disfluency are linked by a curved line.

Prolongations

Prolongations are the second primary characteristic of stuttering considered in the profile. As with repetitions they are recorded from the 100 word sample, and are entered in the profile according to the target phoneme which is prolonged. There is a further subdivision of prolongations into those which are audible and those which are inaudible and also whether the prolongation is heard as greater in duration than 1 sec. The 1 sec. duration has been suggested as a relevant cut-off in the assessment of disfluency by a number of authors (e.g. Van Riper 1982). It is suggested that prolongations greater than 1 sec. are indications of severe disfluency and are often accompanied by increased muscular tension.

The location of the prolongation is recorded under the same format as that for repetitions noting position within the tone unit (head, nucleus or tail) whether occurring on a stressed or unstressed syllable, and location within the word, phrase and clause as appropriate. Audible prolongations are grouped according to manner of production and the individual target phonemes. Silent prolongations mainly involve the closure phase of stops and are further subdivided into place of articulation: labial, alveolar, velar and other. They may be accompanied by glottal closure but this phonetic detail is not coded in the profile.

For both silent and audible prolongations, the presence of oscillations of the vocal folds or supraglottal articulatory organs is indicated where relevant. The criteria used for charting the location of the prolongations are the same as for repetitions, and totals for the type, the relative duration and the location can all easily be obtained from the chart (see Fig. 7 and Appendix).

Pauses

It is possible to chart the type, frequency and location of pauses using similar criteria to those used for repetitions and prolongations. However, the inclusion of pauses in any assessment of stuttering does present a number of special problems. Firstly, in a primarily auditorily based profiling scheme such as this it is difficult in many cases to differentiate between an unfilled pause, defined as a detectable gap in the acoustic signal and a silent prolongation. Secondly, pauses in themselves, in contrast to long prolongations and multiple elemental or syllabic repetitions are not so obviously characteristic features of stuttering, as they occur frequently in normal speech and serve a variety of functions (see discussion in chapter 3). Pausing patterns may however be useful indications of a pathological disfluency when for example pauses occur in abnormal positions e.g. within words, or when they are abnormally long or abnormally frequent. Unfortunately there are at present no adequate normative data on the location, frequency and type of pause in normal speech so it is difficult to devise suitable criteria for charting them in the profile. However, using similar principles as described above for repetitions and prolongations, a tentative profiling chart for pauses is included as Section 3 of the profile (Fig. 8).

Pauses are first logged according to type: "filled" e.g. "um", "er" etc. or "unfilled" e.g. silent intervals. As mentioned above, where a silent interval appears to comprise an inaudible prolongation (e.g. the closure phase of a stop) this is logged under prolongations. Similarly where a pause occurs between individual reiterations in a repetition instance, this is coded as a slow repetition.

The pauses are then located, as with prolongations and repetitions, at the prosodic, the lexical, the phrasal and the clause level. At the prosodic level they are entered as appearing during the head, immediately prior to or just after the nuclear syllable (PRE or POST) during the tail, or at the tone unit boundary. Under the phrasal level, the pause is entered if it occurs within the phrase, e.g. between a determiner and noun in a noun phrase. If the pause occurs during a word the appropriate lexical item in the phrase is underlined. At the clause level, the location of the pause is marked with a – in the relevant place in the constituent structure.

Discussion of a sample profile

To illustrate the use of the profiling scheme outlined in this chapter, the three sections of a sample profile of a stutterer are included in the Appendix. The speaker has been identified by his therapist as a severe stutterer. His conversational speech is transcribed phonetically in the first part of the Appendix. For the purposes of the profile we have taken the first 100 words of the sample text and transcribed it using the appropriate coding conventions discussed above.

Observation of the profile charts illustrates the distinctive characteristics of this speaker. Regarding the repetitions and prolongations (Sections 1 and 2) the figures at the bottom right of each chart show the total number of disfluencies for this sample (11 repetitions and 24 prolongations). Most of the prolongations were perceptually longer than 1 sec. and tended to be linked to the closure phase of stops (the labial place of articulation predominating). We can hypothesize that muscular tension is relatively high during these prolongations, although we have not measured tension directly. Clues lie in the relatively forceful release of stops, such as the /k/ and medial /t/ in "accountant" and the extreme length of some of the prolongations. Increased tension also appears to be present in most of the repetitions, which are coded as slow repetitions. We suggest that the differentiation of prolongations and repetitions in this profile into the two basic types (greater or less than 1 sec. for prolongations, slow versus normal for repetitions) offers a means of quantifying severity of stuttering, which is not readily available from traditional methods, such as for example those based on disfluency counts.

The profile shows also that the prolongations tended to occur on the nuclear syllable in the tone unit and were slightly more likely to occur on stressed syllables rather than unstressed. Repetitions, however, showed quite different patterns. They were mainly single word repetitions (one reiteration per stuttering instance) and these tended to be unstressed words belonging to the grammatical "function" word class such as coordinators, copulars, determiners etc, occurring relatively early in the tone unit, in the head.

Observation of the lexical level data reveals that the majority of prolongations and elemental repetitions occurred word initially. If they occurred word internally then in all cases but one they occurred in syllable initial position. The grammatical analysis revealed that prolongations occurred mainly on nouns, verbs and adjectives with the majority occurring on the verbal or post-verbal constituent (11 occurred on the O or C element, 4 on the V, and 2 on the post-verbal A). The subject element of the clause was involved only twice (for one repetition and one prolongation).

In view of the general difficulties in profiling pauses indicated above, only filled pauses are coded here under Section 3. Of the ten such pauses identified in this sample, 6 occurred in the head of the tone unit, and two just prior to the nucleus. All except one occurred within a phrase, which we suggest is probably an abnormal distribution and may be characteristic of disfluency. At the clause level the analysis showed all except 2 occurred in the post-verbal O element, which follows the trend exemplified by the prolongations.

Further developments

In this chapter we have discussed a profiling procedure which should be a potentially useful tool for both research and therapy for it permits a considerable amount of relevant phonetic, prosodic and syntactic information to be portrayed. When used in conjunction with global quantitative measures such as those suggested by Costello and Ingham (1984) including percentage of syllables stuttered, duration of stuttering episodes, rate of speech length of stutter-free utterances and speech quality it will give considerably more information than traditional assessment procedures. Clinically, the predominance of one type of disfluency could have important implications suggesting the type of therapy that might be most suitable for a particular speaker. The types of location might also suggest to the therapist the most suitable material to be used at various stages of therapy. Finally the detail in the profile and the quantitative measures would provide sensitive measurement of progress. The profile would indicate, for example, that a client had reduced the length of each repetition or prolongation although overall the number of instances of repetitions had remained the same. Similarly a shift of disfluent behaviour, for example tending to repeat elements rather than single words, would also be readily seen on this profile.

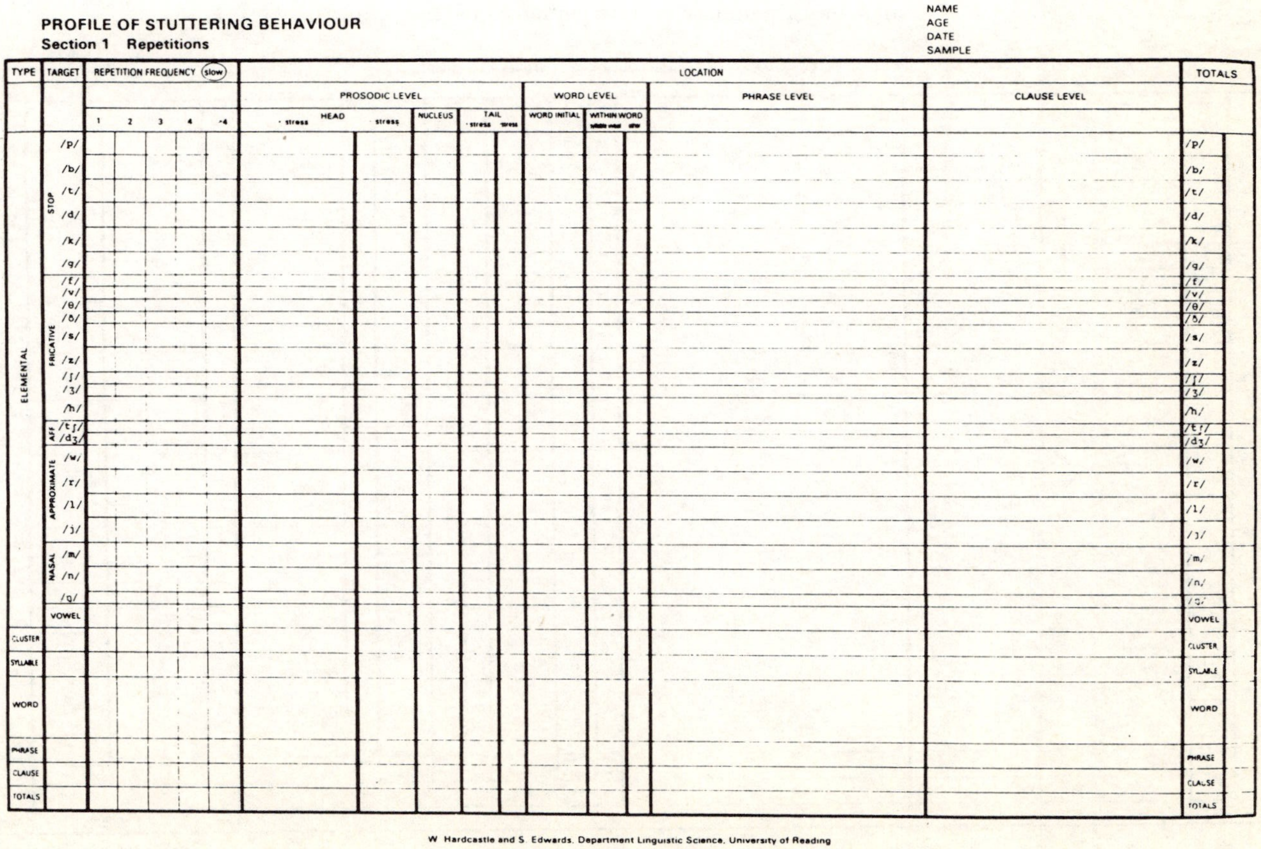

Fig. 6. Chart: Profile of stuttering behaviour. Section 1 Repetitions

PROFILE OF STUTTERING BEHAVIOUR
Section 2 Prolongations

NAME
AGE
DATE
SAMPLE

TYPE	TARGET		DURATION		+osc	LOCATION										TOTALS	
						PROSODIC LEVEL					WORD LEVEL			PHRASE LEVEL	CLAUSE LEVEL		
						HEAD		NUCLEUS	TAIL		WORD INITIAL	WITHIN WORD					
			<1 sec	>1 sec		-stress	stress		-stress	stress		[illegible]	other				
AUDIBLE	+ VOICE STOP CLOSURE	/b/														/b/	
		/d/														/d/	
		/g/														/g/	
	- VOICE FRICATIVE	/f/														/f/	
		/θ/														/θ/	
		/s/														/s/	
		/ʃ/														/ʃ/	
		/h/														/h/	
	+ VOICE FRICATIVE	/v/														/v/	
		/ð/														/ð/	
		/z/														/z/	
		/ʒ/														/ʒ/	
	VOICE AFF	/dʒ/															
	APPROXIMATE	/w/														/w/	
		/ɹ/														/ɹ/	
		/j/														/j/	
		/l/														/l/	
	NASAL	/m/														/m/	
		/n/														/n/	
		/ŋ/														/ŋ/	
	VOWEL															VOWEL	
SILENT	STOP CLOSURE	LAB														LAB	
		ALV														ALV	
		VEL														VEL	
	OTHER															OTHER	
	TOTALS															TOTALS	

W Hardcastle and S Edwards, Department Linguistic Science, University of Reading

Fig. 7. Chart: Profile of stuttering behaviour, Section 2 Prolongations

NAME:
AGE:
DATE:
SAMPLE:

PROFILE OF STUTTERING BEHAVIOUR

Section 3   Pauses

TYPE		LOCATION						
		Prosodic Level				Phrase Level	Clause Level	
Filled	Unfilled	Head	Nucleus Pre Post	Tail	Boundary	Within Phrase	Within Clause	Boundary

Fig. 8. Chart: Profile of stuttering behaviour, Section 3 Pauses

5

Stuttering: theories as to its nature and cause

Most modern writers on the subject of stuttering emphasize the complexity of its manifestations, the inconclusive findings of research into its nature and, above all, the mystery surrounding its etiology. On the one hand it is possible to find subjects to fit almost any theory, and, on the other, no theory seems to relate successfully to each of even the smallest number of stutterers presenting for treatment in an unselected group. It has been said that the only common denominator distinguishing those who stutter from those who do not is 'the fact of stuttering' (Perkins 1965, 17). But since no two stutterers are alike in either the overt symptoms or the complex of attitudes revealed towards communication, even this is in some doubt.

As has already been suggested, the distinction between 'normal' nonfluency and the disorder called stuttering is far from clear. Parents are usually the first to make a diagnosis, and Johnson and his associates (1959), Bloodstein, Alper and Zisk (1965) and others have pointed out the variability in judgements at this stage among those closely involved with children. For many speech therapists and other workers in this area, the point at which early nonfluencies may be regarded as stuttering and therefore to be 'treated', however indirectly, is equally ill-defined.

At a later stage in its development, a severe stutter will be confidently named as such by professional worker and layman alike. But how are we to relate the rapid repetitions and vocalized interruptions of one speaker, the slow blocking behaviour of another and the apparently fluent performance of a third, so skilful in substituting for feared words and circumlocuting every difficulty that little or no disruption occurs? The last will feel himself to be as much a stutterer as the other two, although those round him may be unaware of any problem. He may, in fact, be far more 'fluent' than many whose speech is marked by pauses, filled and unfilled, repetitions and interruptions (see chapter 3), but who neither consider themselves nor are considered to stutter. (The great variety in both the outward manifestations of stuttering and the emotional aspects of anticipation and reaction will be discussed in more detail in chapters 6 and 7).

An attempt will be made in this chapter to survey the main etiological and other theories, but two points should perhaps be made here. As Beech and Fransella (1968) have emphasized, 'There is, as yet, no hard evidence as to whether or not "stuttering" can be regarded as a unitary phenomenon.' As long ago as 1889 Ssikorski questioned whether stuttering 'is a single disorder or a number of disorders which have been grouped together because they have been insufficiently analyzed'. In his chapter on 'types of stutterers' from which this quotation was taken, Van Riper (1971) discusses various attempts that have been made to classify stutterers into groups and subgroups. And while schemes such as Robinson's

(1964, 100–101), describing four common patterns of clinical problems, have been found useful by many clinicians, a great deal more research is needed before our ideas about the existence of discrete 'types' can be developed into a truly useful therapeutic tool.

The second important point to be made is that while the question most frequently asked about stuttering is 'What is the cause?' the most typically held belief, amongst therapists at least, is that any one example of this disorder has developed not from a single cause, but as the result of 'a complex interrelationship between many factors' (Andrews and Harris 1964, 16). And this is the view to which we subscribe.

The literature on theories of stuttering runs into volumes and our survey can only be brief. We shall try to cover only the more recent ideas, specifically as they still influence current thinking and therapy. (In his excellent and comprehensive study *The nature of stuttering* (1971), Van Riper traces the historical development of the main theories in chapters 11–14.) We have grouped them, rather loosely, under the headings 'organic', including some of the studies of possible physical or constitutional factors, 'psychogenic', where personality traits and, particularly, neurotic features are given most weight, 'learned behaviour', in which anticipation and conflict are seen as the key, and 'evaluational', where the diagnosis of the parents plays a major role.

Some organic theories of stuttering

Since it is the physical aspect of stuttering that is the most immediately striking to the observer, it is not surprising that many attempts have been made to find an organic or constitutional factor as the basis of the disorder. A number of studies have suggested strongly that a genetic element exists, as stutterers have been shown to have more stutterers in their families than non-stutterers. Beech and Fransella (1968), in their careful survey of the research on genetic and organic factors, are inclined to this view, as are Andrews and Harris (1964), and many others. But, as we shall see, Johnson (1959) maintains that the adult's expectations and attitudes are more responsible than any genetic possibility for the recurrence of stuttering in families. It would seem, on balance, that something, as yet undiscovered, may be inherited—a tendency for developing speech to be vulnerable to disruption—and that psychological and environmental factors play their part in precipitating this vulnerability into disorder and perpetuating it.

The search for an organic abnormality within the central nervous system has led people to investigate the cerebral dominance of stutterers, their EEG records, possible links with epilepsy, general motor abilities and even eye movements. Beech and Fransella review these findings as well as those related to metabolism and the cardiovascular system. Their conclusions are cautious. They suggest from the evidence that 'the stutterer may have incomplete cerebral dominance or bilateral representation of speech' (103). A more recent experiment, outlined by Dorman and Porter (1975), however, refutes even this tentative suggestion. Beech and Fransella state that the stutterer *could* have 'some minimal disorder of the central nervous system' (104). But they emphasize that this is by no means clearly demonstrated. In other areas they find a mass of conflicting evidence, as does Van Riper in his review of 'organicity and stuttering' (1971, ch. 13). Full discussion of these ideas can be found in these two works, and Perkins, in his contribution to Sheehan, 1970, presents an interesting analysis of physiological studies and asks some very pertinent questions in his concluding section on 'new directions'. All agree that many questions on the organic side remain unanswered and suggest the need for more thorough research.

Of the more recent theories, one which has aroused a great deal of interest and actually given birth to a systematic form of treatment is that concerning impaired auditory feedback. The constitutional difference suggested here is not so much in organic make-up as in the functioning of the auditory monitoring system for sequential speech (see chapter 2). Since 1951, when Lee first described how normal fluency could be disturbed by playing back the speaker's utterance to him with one-fifteenth to one-tenth of a second's delay (Delayed Auditory Feedback), there has been a good deal of attention given to the possible connection between auditory feedback and stuttering. Here as always, however, evidence and opinions conflict. Normal speakers have been found to vary in their responses to DAF. The disfluency produced by them is said by some to be different in nature from stuttering. However, various experiments in blocking out or 'masking' auditory feedback while the stutterer is speaking have shown some striking results. Cherry and Sayers (1956) found that disfluency was almost completely eliminated when very loud noise excluded both air and bone conduction of sounds. When air conduction only was masked, little effect was produced. They concluded therefore that stuttering might be the result of faulty bone-conduction feedback. As it is the low frequencies that are transmitted by bone conduction, they experimented further by masking out low frequencies. Here they found more individual variation amongst stutterers' responses, but, in general, the results showed an increase in fluency.

Later, experiments began on the effects of the deliberate delay of auditory feedback in stutterers. Some of them reacted in the same way as normal speakers, others, especially the more severe, became more, not less fluent. In several studies the delay time was varied until the 'optimum' delay was found, under which conditions disfluency was much reduced or eliminated. Soderberg (1959), Bohr (1963) and Goldiamond (1965) describe just some examples of a wide range of experimentation. Several workers found that DAF, while not eliminating stuttering, helped the speaker to stutter in a more relaxed way—easy repetitions and prolongations of sound were produced instead of hard blocks. Soderberg (1968), Goldiamond and others used DAF to produce a slow 'prolonged' speech pattern to replace stuttering, which could gradually be modified towards normal speed of utterance. In his 1969 paper, Soderberg reviews the studies of DAF so far and points out a number of factors needing further investigation including the severity of the stuttering involved, delay time and intensity of feedback.

Researchers have continued to study the effects both of masking with noise and of DAF. Two main explanations for the reduction of disfluency in the presence of auditory masking have been put forward. One is that anxiety is reduced through the stutterer's inability to hear his disfluencies and therefore they decrease. The other is that it is the resultant 'modified vocalization' (Wingate 1970), which reduces disfluency: that is, speakers were found to increase vocal intensity and to slow down the rate of utterance under these conditions. Several later studies, e.g. Adams and Moore 1972 and Adams and Hutchinson 1974, provide strong support for this latter theory. It should also be noted that the nonfluencies of normal speakers were found to be reduced by masking (Silverman and Goodban 1972).

Just why DAF should reduce disfluency in many stutterers when it produces it in normal speakers is still not fully explained. Watts (1973) suggests two main possibilities. The first is that the stutterer 'tunes out' and therefore is cut off from the feedback of his disfluencies, as with masking. The second proposes that it is the prolongation of speech used to adapt to the delay which produces the fluency. That both fluent speakers and stutterers react to 'noise' and DAF in a number of different ways is clear. Why they do so is not. Whether or not a number of stutterers do suffer a disturbance of auditory feedback is still debated. The 'prolonged speech' technique evolved from DAF, like most techniques used in therapy, seems to be of great value to some stutterers and of little use to others. And, as we shall see (chapter 7), it shares with other techniques the same problem in its use outside the clinical situation. In stress situations particularly, many stutterers find it difficult to use any alternative to their habitual speech pattern.

In his chapter on stuttering as a result of disturbed feedback, Van Riper (1971, 393–6) discusses the part played by proprioception and the tactile sense in the monitoring of speech (see also chapter 2 above). He postulates that although as infants we rely initially on auditory feedback to check our utterance, 'it would be too burdensome if we always had to play our speech by ear—if we were eternally doomed to listen to each sound and syllable of each word to ensure its correctness'. He believes that as soon as the motor sequences involved in word production seem to be able to be produced correctly without constant auditory scrutiny, the major responsibility for the monitoring of speech is passed over to the 'kinaesthetic-tactual-proprioceptive' information processing system. He suggests that the change-over takes place gradually and probably intermittently at first, and that in some children it is this period of change which is the vulnerable one. 'For some time there may be some interference between the auditory and proprioceptive signals which could lead to broken words. Or there may be over-load.' He does not find it surprising either that children should begin to stutter at this stage or even that most children should show some disfluency. 'Over-loaded circuits oscillate and jam. Once the monitoring of the motoric sequencing of words can be turned over to proprioception, much of this over-load is reduced. Auditory interference no longer has much impact.'

Van Riper believes that normally fluent adults use this system, which he terms 'somesthesia', as their primary one. A stutterer subjected to auditory masking is forced to do the same, which is another explanation for his greater fluency—he has created a barrier against any auditory interference or distortion which might be present. Van Riper also draws our attention to the fact that many stutterers seem able to speak fluently while whispering or pantomiming speech. He concludes that it seems highly plausible that distortion in the total feedback system may be responsible for disfluency: 'The distortion may reside in the auditory signals alone and be introduced by bilateral phase differences between bone- and air-conducted sidetone or in interference produced by auditory and proprioceptive competition or in overload, or in the central processing of information.' He feels, with others, that this area, which we are just beginning to explore, will teach us much about the essential nature of stuttering. The role of different feedback mechanisms in speech production has received some attention recently in the phonetic literature (e.g. Ringel and Steer 1963, Scott and Ringel 1971, Gammon *et al.* 1971, Horii *et al.* 1973, Hardcastle 1975).

The main problem in considering any of the organic possibilities as a cause of stuttering would seem to lie in the periods of fluency experienced by most stutterers. These may last for minutes, hours, days or even weeks. If there is a constitutional factor at work, why is it not at work the whole time? West's theory of a link with epilepsy (1958) makes some sense of the intermittent recurrence of most forms of stuttering, but he himself presents his view as speculation and, so far, no evidence has been found to support it. It could be said that the organic factor needs something else to trigger it off such as anxiety or excessive tension. But despite the obvious relationship between moments of anxiety and the production of muscular tension in some stuttered speech, observation of the behaviour of many stutterers, especially young children, suggests that their disfluencies very frequently occur when they appear to experience no anxiety at all. Many adult stutterers have also acknowledged this. The emotional reaction may *follow* a block or a series of disfluencies, but is by no means invariably the cause. Only for the relatively small group of severe, consistent stutterers does a mainly organic origin seem a real possibility.

Some psychogenic theories of stuttering

In discussing some of the ideas related to psychogenic theories of stuttering, we come up against the question of whether the inevitable psychological components of most developed stuttering arise in reaction to disfluency or have been a part of the problem since its onset. Often the assumption is made that, since older children and adult stutterers may experience anxiety, frustration, anger and even withdrawal in the face of many speaking situations, a psychological state producing negative emotions of this kind must lie at the basis of the disorder. However, in chapter 6 we shall show how it is the increase in emotional reaction and avoidance which, in the main, distinguishes advanced from early stuttering; that is, as secondary characteristics to the disfluency itself. Therapists will have observed an extraordinary lack of concern in many younger stutterers, sometimes despite severe speech disruption. Much of the work in favour of psychogenic theory, which is anyway inconclusive, would seem to be invalidated, since adult subjects have been used. It is clearly of great importance in therapy to pay as much attention to the psychological aspects of stuttering as to the physical symptoms. But though these undoubtedly exacerbate and perpetuate the problem, they may be seen in most cases as the result rather than the cause of disfluency.

Workers in this area have looked into the personality rather than the physical make-up of stutterers in their search for specific characteristics which might set them apart from normal speakers. Beech and Fransella (1968, 124) have made an excellent survey of many of these investigations and draw some clear and some less definite conclusions. From the evidence they find that there is nothing to suggest that the stutterer 'has a particular type of personality or group of traits that differentiates him from the non-stutterer'. Further, 'there is little unequivocal evidence that stutterers as a group are more neurotic or maladjusted than non-stutterers'. They do suggest that they may be less ready to accept themselves as they are and 'appear to have a higher general level of anxiety than non-stutterers'. Neither of these points would seem to stand as a firm basis for a psychogenic diagnosis. Sheehan's review of 'Personality approaches' (1970, ch. 3) is a very comprehensive one, including the use of Rorschach, TAT, Self-Concept, MMPI, intelligence studies and many others. He too concludes that stutterers do not show a common personality pattern and that in group studies, stutterers 'cannot be distinguished from normal-speaking controls' (131).

In any group of human beings a proportion of them will suffer from neuroses of every kind. Stutterers are no exception. Most of us display neurotic behaviour at some time. Again, stutterers are no exception. And in view of the enormous problems many of them face in trying to communicate, it is only surprising that more of them are not maladjusted in this speech-oriented culture of ours.

Yet, for over a century, stuttering has been many times labelled a psychoneurosis. Coriat (1927, 1931, 1943) was perhaps the most lucid of those who expressed the disorder in psychoanalytic terms. For him, it was the result of oral fixation. For others (Fenichel 1945, Heilpern 1941) the fixation was believed to be at the anal stage of development. Stein (1953) saw the stutterer as having a compulsion neurosis. In moments of anxiety he regresses to the babbling stage of speech, reflected in his repetitions, while prolongations are regarded as expressions of aggression. Glauber (1958) sees the conflict between the id and the super-ego as the root of the problem, while Barbara (1965, 160) sees the stutterer as 'suffering from unhealthy relationships and neurotic difficulties, which become expressed overtly when he speaks and especially so at the moment of stuttering'. He, at least, does not view the problem as the province of the analyst alone. He recommends a team approach which includes 'the skills and orientation of a speech therapist and the skills and orientation of a psychotherapist'. Sheehan (1970, 132) is in agreement here: 'Though stutterers do not need psychotherapy just because they are stutterers, they seem to profit from a program integrating psychotherapy with speech therapy.' Many therapists experienced in this field would undoubtedly agree that such an approach would be ideal for a number of their clients.

Strictly psychoanalytic theories of the nature and cause of stuttering (and those mentioned are a small sample) do little to enlighten us, since they have yet to produce any evidence that can be weighed. Other theories, however, shortly to be discussed, to do with 'conflict'—not between different aspects of the personality and its development, but in relation to the act of speaking itself—overlap to some extent with this psychogenic group, in their emphasis on psychological factors.

Stuttering as learned behaviour

It is impossible in this brief survey to go into the learning theories which influence many of the current theories of stuttering. In a closely reasoned chapter, Van Riper (1971, ch. 12) discusses the development of these ideas from studies of operant and classical conditioning. The 'consistency effect', defined by Van Riper as 'the tendency of stuttering to occur repeatedly in the same situations and on the same words', is put forward by some as clear evidence that stuttering behaviour is 'learned'. Equally, the seemingly contradictory phenomenon of 'adaptation'—the ability of most stutterers to become more fluent in successive readings of the same passage—is seen as supporting learned behaviour theory. Sheehan (1958, 132) explains this fact as follows: 'The stuttering which occurs during the first reading decreases fear sufficiently to permit less stuttering on the second; that which occurs during the second reading reduces fear further so that there is less stuttering on the third etc.' But since there is evidence that non-stutterers also become progressively more fluent in successive readings (Williams, Silverman and Kools 1968), the two groups of speakers cannot be said to be differentiated by the adaptation effect. The well-documented fact that most adult stutterers can predict very accurately when and on what they will stutter forms the basis of several of the more developed ideas. Yet Silverman and Williams (1972) found that in a group of eighty-four stutterers between the ages of 8 and 16 years, over half failed to predict the majority of their stuttering, the older ones not being significantly more accurate than the younger ones. At what point this ability to predict develops and forms a trigger for particular moments of stuttering is not clear. All the more interesting theories throw light on the way in which a stutter, once begun, develops into a habitual pattern of behaviour. None of them, however, explains entirely satisfactorily how and why it begins in the first place.

Both Van Riper and Beech and Fransella select Wischner's theory of 'expectancy' as one of this group worthy of consideration and further research. In experiments and papers produced between 1947 and 1969, Wischner has expanded his basic premise that certain words and situations produce anxiety, causing the speaker to stutter. The disfluency having occurred, anxiety is reduced and thus the stuttering behaviour is reinforced. Like Johnson, Wischner believes that it is the disapproval or anxiety of the parents in relation to normal nonfluency which sets up the reaction of anxiety in the child. From then on, delaying and avoidance behaviours are developed to escape the 'punishment' of unfavourable reactions from others. While accepting Wischner's idea that avoidance behaviours do often decrease anxiety and therefore themselves become reinforced as part of the pattern, Van Riper points out that these behaviours may appear even more abnormal to the listener than the expected stuttering, and receive an even stronger punishing reaction. As a stutterer himself, he speaks feelingly of the punishment experienced from the sheer frustration involved, which must surely become greater as the stuttering event becomes more prolonged and complex.

Joseph Sheehan has outlined his 'conflict' theory of stuttering in Eisenson's symposium on stuttering (1958) and elsewhere. To him and his colleagues it is an approach/avoidance conflict—that between the need to speak and the desire to remain silent, with a further conflict between the wish for silence and the fear of it. He too points to parental disapproval as the originator of the conflict, producing the 'guilt' about speech failure to struggle against a child's natural desire to express himself. We cannot go into Sheehan's highly complicated experimental work here, concerning the role of the disfluency itself as a fear-reducer, or that of the avoidance behaviour as a tension-producer. But it forms the basis of his therapeutic approach (to be dealt with more fully in chapter 7) where the stutterer is urged to stutter openly, and to discard 'false fluency' gained by avoidance of stuttering. By 1970 Sheehan had developed his ideas into a 'role-conflict' theory: 'a disorder of the social presentation of the self . . . not a speech disorder, but a conflict revolving around self and role, an identity problem' (4). He outlines his theory in his recent book on research and therapy (1970), taking as his basis the fact that most stutterers are disfluent only in certain situations or 'roles'.

While these writers join with the group we shall consider next in seeing the reactions of a child's listeners as crucial to the development of the disorder, they do not pursue the link between normal nonfluency and the onset of stuttering. Nor do they suggest any reason why some children are more vulnerable to conflict through parental disapproval than others, when many a non-stutterer must have been subject to the same pressures and corrections. They do not go into the question of why one group of children should 'learn' these abnormal behaviours while others do not.

The role of evaluation in the onset of stuttering

Wendell Johnson was probably the first to focus attention on the powerful effects of labelling a child a stutterer. In a report (1959) of research stretching from 1934 to 1957, he concludes that 'at the point of origin of the problem of stuttering the most crucial single factor to be considered is that of the listener's sensitivity to the speaker's nonfluencies, his inclination to evaluate them as undesirable and distressing and particularly his tendency to classify them specifically as "stuttering" '. His theory is that, while all children pass through a stage of normal nonfluency in the development of speech, some authority figures, usually the parents, are more inclined to be disturbed by this fact than others, to react to it unfavourably, to transmit this reaction to the child and cause him to become aware that he is doing something unacceptable when he speaks. This, Johnson maintains, is the point at which the child begins to produce truly abnormal speech behaviour—when, in fact, he begins to 'stutter', in order to avoid the unwanted disfluencies.

His hypothesis is concerned with the interaction between speaker and listener, and he shows how the judgement of the 'primary' listener, usually the mother, will affect other listeners in the child's environment: they will hear what she hears. He discusses three major variables in the development of this situation. The first is the listener's sensitivity to the speaker's nonfluency, which would be heightened, for instance, where the listener or any of the family is a stutterer; the second, 'the speaker's degree of nonfluency as objectively determined' and the third, 'the speaker's sensitivity to his own nonfluency and to the listener's evaluative reactions to his nonfluency'.

Johnson's report covers in great detail factors such as types of disfluency classified as stuttering, the listener's perceptual set, which influences his judgement, the listener's sense of fluency norms, and so on. He found that the degree of the speaker's nonfluency and his sensitivity to these nonfluencies were less important than listener evaluation at first, but later contributed more and more, once he had been made to perceive himself as 'a stutterer'.

There can be no doubt that parental anxiety and parental correction plays its part in the development of stuttering in many children. For that reason, the basis of therapy with the very young child always seeks to reduce this anxiety and to prevent correction. The aim is to keep the child unaware of disfluency or at least to prevent the build-up of guilt about it. However, more work needs to be done to extend the evidence in favour of Johnson's theory, since it has yet to be proved that all stutterers have been the object of anxiety and criticism in their early childhood. Although the memories of adult stutterers may not necessarily be relied upon, of 186 clients treated intensively at the Speech Therapy Unit of the City Literary Institute in London, only eleven of them related the onset of their stutter to the reactions of their parents; and when asked about their parents' attitude to their disfluency as children, most of them said that they 'ignored it' or were 'understanding', implying either absence of criticism or positive support.

Oliver Bloodstein has studied the phenomena of stuttering over a long period and written many papers on the subject. One contribution to Barbara 1965, produced with colleagues Alper and Zisk, concerns 'Stuttering as an outgrowth of normal disfluency'—clearly in agreement with Johnson's theory in many respects. We shall be dealing more fully with 'normal' nonfluency in the next chapter; but they see the relationship of the two as crucial to any discussion about the onset of the disorder. Finding that the consistency effect (described above) was also present in some features of normal nonfluency (i.e. repetitions of syllables and words) they concluded that non-stuttering children, too, experience some anticipatory reaction to speech and that the difference between the two groups of children is a matter of degree. Referring back to Bloodstein 1961, they quote: 'The only distinction which one can validly make appears to be a purely relative one between struggle reactions which are mild and occasional and those which are more severe and persistent' (40).

They point to other aspects of speech besides fluency which might cause a child to anticipate difficulty: errors of articulation, inadequate language and, at a very crucial time for the 'diagnosis' of stuttering, reading difficulty on starting school. These features are often sources of anxiety to parents. Bloodstein et al. emphasize, with Johnson, that 'there appears to be a decided overlap between the kinds of speech hesitancy which are described by parents of stutterers as the earliest symptoms of "stuttering", and the descriptions of early speech hesitations which are given by parents of children who speak "normally"' (51). In conclusion, they find a 'basic implausibility about any conception of human behaviour which separates people in an unqualified way into "normal" and "abnormal"'. Bloodstein (1970) examines further this 'continuity hypothesis' and we shall return to it in the next chapter.

This brief survey of some of the theories of stuttering cannot be considered comprehensive, but it is to be hoped that it provides some impression of the scope of work done in this area. As most writers on the subject have concluded, more careful research is needed to extend our knowledge in many directions. We cannot, surely, expect that at last 'a cause' will be discovered, but if further investigation can teach us more of what lies behind some of the forms and features of stuttering and help in its alleviation, time and effort will not be wasted.

Popular concepts concerning the cause of stuttering

Since we are concerned in this volume with the effects of stuttering on communication, we should perhaps take equal note of the views of the communicators themselves as to the nature and cause of the disorder. It is, after all, those who come into contact with stutterers in everyday life and the stutterers themselves, not the 'authorities' on stuttering, who largely produce the climate of opinion and reaction in which disfluency is actually experienced. They, the speakers and listeners, may view stuttering as an 'affliction' to be pitied or ridiculed or simply regard it as one aspect of a person's behaviour of little significance. Some people, of course, with a relative or friend who stutters, will have taken the trouble to read about the problem and their view will probably be influenced by some of the ideas already discussed. Many stutterers have read and considered various theories at great length and, more often than not, are none the wiser. We are concerned here, however, with general views, whatever their source, since these are what govern some of the attitudes affecting communication situations for all concerned.

Reactions to stuttering from strangers vary as much as reactions to other 'abnormalities' of behaviour. Depending on both the knowledge and personality of the listener, as well as the attitude of the stutterer to his own difficulty, there may be impatience, pity, alarm, protectiveness or, most commonly, plain embarrassment. Children sent out to confront the general public with their disfluency, in this country at least, seem to be treated on the whole with patience and sympathy. This may not be so when the listener is in a hurry or easily alarmed, but most of the children sent out during intensive courses at the School for the Study of the Disorders of Human Communication at Blackfriars in London, for instance, report back favourably. With adults, this is not so often the case. Embarrassment seems to be more frequent, as does impatience, especially in situations where others may be waiting, such as queues for tickets or in crowded shops or pubs. These are our observations from accompanying stutterers on outside 'assignments', and the point should be made that they themselves often exaggerate the strength of any reaction.

The severity and type of stuttering naturally to some extent governs the degree of listener reaction. Mild disfluency will often pass unnoticed. It appears that the most difficult manifestation for the listener to contend with is the silent block at the beginning of an utterance, where the speaker stands rooted to the spot and the listener is similarly immobilized—that and the loud preliminary repetition or interpolated sound, especially where there is severe facial contortion. Once the stutterer can begin, the tension is reduced on both sides. While not going all the way with Sheehan (1970) in his belief that the stutterer should go out and stutter to all and sundry, seeking out every opportunity to display his disfluency, we have found that those who learn to stutter without shame, looking their listener in the eye and remaining calm, have reported far less unfavourable reaction. It seems, basically, that the listener needs reassurance that the speaker is in command of himself.

It is this point, too, which has its effect on the stutterer's contact with people he meets more often—at work or socially. On the whole, the more the stutterer is known to others as 'normal' apart from his speech difficulty and the more accustomed the listener becomes to the disfluent speech, the less adverse reaction there is. But where the stutterer himself remains desperately anxious every time he has to communicate with someone and cuts himself off from speaking situations, those round him stay on their guard, often avoid conversation with him and complete the vicious circle of isolation. With the exception of people particularly easily threatened by something they do not understand, the more the stutterer takes his disfluency in his stride, the more his listeners will do so.

From questioning members of the public, we have found that people who know a stutterer as a friend or relative may not have a very clear view as to the nature or cause of the problem, but will tend to base any judgement they have on the example they are familiar with. If their stutterer fell down the stairs at three years, they will assume (if they have made no further investigation) that some such incident causes stuttering. If their friend or relative is anxious and withdrawn, the cause is thought to be 'nerves' or 'psychological'. Where there is no familiarity with a person who stutters, opinions and attitudes may be handed down from what Johnson refers to as 'folklore', or gleaned from articles in magazines or newspapers. A kindly woman keeping house for a group of adult stutterers on a working holiday in Devon commented to the therapist with amazement 'But they look so well!' In her mind presumably was the expectation that her guests would be suffering from some illness. The oft-quoted list of famous historical figures or current entertainers who have stuttered is probably partly responsible for the impression in some that stutterers are particularly gifted people.

The important point about the opinions (if any) of the general public about stuttering is the effect they will have on their attitudes towards stutterers. The reactions of the listener, whether they be sympathetic or critical, are as much a part of communication as the utterance of the speaker. Some stutterers are more dependent than others on a favourable reception, but most have increased difficulty in the face of impatience or outright rejection. When asked in a questionnaire 'What reactions to your stutter do you dislike most from the listener?' the overwhelming majority who have attended courses at the City Literary Institute have written such things as 'looking away', 'being embarrassed' or 'impatience'. (No suggestions were given them.) While the question 'What do you find the most helpful reactions to your stutter?' has typically produced replies such as 'when people just listen patiently', 'real interest in what I am saying', 'patience–tolerance'. Most of them imply a need for sympathetic attention on the part of the listener, while acknowledging that the other person has to exercise patience. One reaction few adults seem to welcome is pity. Anyone assuming that a stutterer is sick or inadequate may produce a thoroughly undermining, over-protective attitude. One young man returned furious from an outside assignment, when a well-meaning pedestrian had taken him by the arm and led him along, shouting directions as to a child, when he asked the way to Oxford Circus.

Nevertheless, we agree with Sheehan that it is to some extent the responsibility of the stutterers themselves both to cope with unfavourable reactions and to play their part in seeing that the general public is better informed. This kind of initiative seems to be more common in America than in this country. In Britain, more has been written lately in newspapers and magazines, though articles tend to over-emphasize the suffering entailed. Radio and television programmes have included items on stuttering, but so far attempts to persuade various companies to present a full-length documentary on the disorder have failed. One potential producer commented that it did not seem 'visually exciting'. Others appear to feel that viewers might not tolerate stuttering. The need for more information was made abundantly clear by the response to a mention of available treatment in a national newspaper. We had not realized how many people still thought of stuttering in terms of an illness that could be 'cured', until letters poured in from relatives, friends and stutterers themselves, asking for our 'treatment' to be sent by post, in some cases in a plain envelope.

Though the parents of young children with disfluency problems (whose views we will come to shortly) are the most in need of what information we can give them, others in the stutterer's environment can make a substantial contribution to his or her development as a communicator. Teachers figure largely in a child's life, and it is clear from the reports of adults that the attitude of the teacher towards their difficulty, particularly in reading or speaking in front of a class, has done much to help or hinder their progress both at school and socially. With the development of the speech therapy service in this country, there is increasing liaison between therapist and school. There are no 'rules' as to whether it is better for a child to be spared the experience of speaking or reading before others or urged to do everything the others do, despite difficulty. This will vary in each case. But more often now, though not often enough, therapist and teacher can work out the most helpful approach between them. Stories of ridicule and neglect by teachers are very rare but still the stutterer's failure to respond in oral work can be misunderstood as laziness or inattention. Unless the teacher knows that disfluency varies from situation to situation, he or she may well misjudge a child who talks and shouts happily with friends in play and then sits dumb when asked a question in class. Many children and adults have admitted that they have pretended not to know something, rather than attempt a verbal answer.

Following school, the next most crucial period in a stutterer's life is when he tries to get his first job. In some instances, of course, the speech difficulty makes no difference. But where a job entails speaking, particularly to the general public, many employers are chary of taking on a stutterer. He is very often at his worst in the initial interview situation and while he may be quite fluent with friends or when once settled into a situation, he may present himself so unfavourably that the employer rejects him out of hand. In one case, three referees wrote to assure an employer that a particular person had very little trouble in the work he wished to do. Fortunately, the employer took the risk and all was well. Before that, however, the young man had been turned down for many posts over two years of depressing and frustrating job-hunting. Many stutterers settle for work which does not suit them, simply because it entails little or no speech. But we have found that those who have to communicate in their jobs and do not avoid speaking situations, cope with their difficulties far better than those who opt out. Some employers, of course, show great concern for members of their staff and may take great pains to help them to receive treatment. But this is generally when the stutterer's talent or qualifications make him an obvious potential asset to the firm. It is far harder for those employed in jobs without responsibility to get time off to try to improve things. In the present state of general knowledge, most employers cannot really be blamed. It seems high time, however, that stuttering and other speech difficulties were subjects of the same attention and concern as other problems so much more widely discussed and studied by the media now.

Much has been written about the role of parents in the development of a child's stutter and his attitude towards it. And, clearly, the way a parent feels about any aspect of a child's behaviour will have a great influence on how the young person, and indeed later the adult, feels. Many of the parent's attitudes will be governed by what he or she thinks causes the disfluency and what this represents in terms of the expression of psychological or physical defect. Johnson's monumental work already referred to (1959) on the onset of stuttering contains the results of interviews with 600 parents. These were involved in the third of the research programmes described in the book. In Study three, the parents of 150 so-called stuttering children and 150 controls were interviewed. One of the many questions asked was 'What do you think causes stuttering?' The replies were classified under eight headings, with details as given below from Johnson's table pp. 166–7.

1. Physical:
- (*a*) shock to mother
- (*b*) change of handedness
- (*c*) physically inferior speech mechanism
- (*d*) heredity
- (*e*) mental deficiency
- (*f*) birth injury
- (*g*) hearing deficiency
- (*h*) difference in other bodily functions
- (*i*) some illness of the child
- (*j*) being tired
- (*k*) being tickled
- (*l*) because he has cerebral palsy perhaps
- (*m*) polio

2. *Emotional or behavioural:*
   (a)   shock to child
   (b)   inferiority complex
   (c)   pressures of speaking situations
   (d)   carelessness, lack of attention
   (e)   excitement, emotional upset
   (f)   emotional disturbance
   (g)   excitement
   (h)   fear
   (i)   emotional insecurity; being around someone who stutters
   (j)   bad scare
   (k)   too much competition with sibs for attention
   (l)   frustration at table—competing in talking

3. *Nervousness:*
   (a)   nervousness
   (b)   being generally highly strung
   (c)   form of nervous tension

4. *Imitation:*
   (a)   imitation

5. *Discrepancy between talking and thinking:*
   (a)   thinks faster than can talk
   (b)   talks faster than can think
   (c)   inadequate vocabulary
   (d)   immaturity; wants to talk faster than mind works and has inadequate vocabulary, so repeats until he finds the next word
   (e)   talking too fast
   (f)   not thinking before talking
   (g)   talking too fast; can't get one word out so keeps saying it until he can

6. *Handedness:*
   (a)   change of handedness
   (b)   left-handedness
   (c)   lack of cerebral balance

7. *Parental involvement:*
   (a)   punishment of child
   (b)   semantogenic or diagnosogenic factors
   (c)   influenced by conditions in home
   (d)   parental overconcern
   (e)   parents, associates
   (f)   result of father's strictness; got all tied up because tries so hard to say words

8. *'Have no idea':*
   (a)   ? (don't know—have no idea)

This table represents a very wide range of responses. A high percentage of the parents (76 per cent experimental group, 68 per cent control group) expressed some form of belief that the cause of stuttering 'is to be found wholly within the body or personality or behaviour pattern of the speaker'. The most frequently proposed cause under (1), physical, was heredity, while under (2), emotional or behavioural, excitement, emotional upset and emotional disturbance constituted most of the responses. A relatively high number attributed the cause to (3), nervousness, very few to (4), imitation, a comparatively large number to (5), discrepancy between talking and thinking, and very few to (6), handedness. It is interesting to note that only 4 per cent of the parents of the experimental group related the cause to (7), parental involvement, while 16 per cent of the control group did so. Those stating that they had no idea, (8), were 23 per cent of the experimental group and 12 per cent of the control group parents.

Taking just a few of the responses contained in the table, it would seem that a parent's attitude to a child thought to stutter because of 'carelessness' would be very different from that where 'inferiority complex' was suspected as the cause. The first of these is likely to produce a reaction of impatience to the child's disfluency. The second, a phrase most often used inaccurately, is likely to burden the child with a glib, pseudopsychological label, which can follow him into adulthood. Like the child who is called 'shy' or 'doesn't eat', the child diagnosed as having an inferiority complex at some point between the age of 2 years + and 9 years + (the age range of the study) may well find himself compelled to behave accordingly. A mother or father who feels that 'punishment of the child' has caused the problem, will have very different feelings about it from one who relates it to 'thinking faster than he can talk'. In the first case, guilt could produce a wide range of unhelpful reactions, while in the second, there is more likely to be an element of pride in the child's intellectual ability and an attitude that increased maturity will 'sort things out'. These suggestions are sheer speculation, of course, and it would be interesting to try to relate parental behaviour towards disfluency to their ideas about its cause in a properly planned experiment. And, clearly, many other factors besides ideas about causes influence the attitudes of parents and others towards stuttering.

The stutterer's own ideas as to the origins of his difficulty are probably built up from many sources: his parents' ideas, things he has read, the ideas of those who have attempted to help him. He may see it as a 'speech problem', related only to the use of his mechanism, or regard it as indicating some physical or psychological abnormality. Any adult attending courses at the City Literary Institute is asked initially what he believes to be the cause of his stutter. Many express surprise as well as interest when other possibilities besides their own are put forward later in the course of discussion. Like many 'authorities', they often confuse cause with effect. They say they stutter because they 'lack confidence', for instance, labelling themselves in a total way, when, more often than not, it emerges that it is only in certain speech situations that their self-assurance is temporarily at a low ebb. They speak of 'nerves', as if they spend their entire lives in a state of anxiety, and later have to admit that this is not the case. It is just that anxious moments are more readily remembered than carefree ones. We are not trying to minimize the discomfort and apprehension experienced by many who stutter on many occasions, but the exaggeration of this experience in the minds of stutterers and to those who communicate with them can make the task of dealing with the problem in any practical way an even more difficult one.

We have studied the written responses of 186 adult stutterers, attending intensive courses at the City Literary Institute between September 1971 and July 1975, to the question 'What do you believe to be the cause of your stutter?' We find that they can mostly be grouped into Johnson's eight categories and we have attempted to compare the results, bearing in mind that Johnson's responses came from American parents some twenty years ago. Ours are from British stutterers, whose ages range from 18 to 69, but most of whom are in their twenties. We are simply considering the range of ideas expressed and noting those most frequently held. We have added one more category, 'habit', and will also discuss views of 'multiple causes'.

Only eleven could be grouped under (1), physical. Two of these gave 'heredity' as the cause, although as many as 74 reported other members of their families as being stutterers. Five related the onset to early illness or accident causing physical damage, two gave tonsilectomy as the cause, while the other two saw 'tongue-tie' and breathing abnormality respectively as the origin.

Under (2), emotional or behavioural, eleven reported some sort of emotional shock in early childhood. These ranged from being told at the age of three that his mother was dead, to being knocked over by a dog at two and a half years. In addition one spoke of 'attention-seeking', another of 'temper–anger', a third referred to competing with a family of excellent speakers, making fourteen in all.

By far the largest number (apart from those in (8)) come under the general heading of (3), nervousness. Amongst those we have included such statements as 'lack of self-confidence', 'nervous tension', 'nerves' and 'an inestimable degree of shyness'. There were 56 such responses.

(4), (5) and (6) have few supporters. Only three give imitation as the only cause, three relate their problem to discrepancy between talking and thinking and two see a change of handedness as the one significant factor.

Under the heading 'parental involvement', eleven spoke in some way of either parental anxiety about speech or parental pressure to 'speak properly', one of them, alas, adding 'speech therapy at an early age' as a supplementary cause!

Forty-eight stutterers had 'no idea', one of them expressing the matter feelingly with 'God knows! One day I'll write a book about it.' We hope he will. Four simply said 'habit'.

Perhaps the most interesting group, however, were those who set out a number of factors as contributing to their problem. Of these remaining 36, several showed a good deal of insight. One or two are worth quoting:

(1) 'Complex, but probably most influential were divorce of parents when I was two years old. During my early years having two elder sisters who spoke fluently, whilst I was learning to speak. Intense dislike of school. Lack of self-confidence (cause or effect?).'

(2) 'Reinforcement of childish stammer, exacerbated by family history of stammering and later reacting to criticism and suppressing aggression.'
(3) '(a) Fell downstairs at 4 years.
      (b) Forced to change hands.
      (c) Turbulent family life.'

and one rather resounding package deal:

(4) 'Scarlet fever at 3 years.
      Maladjusted childhood.
      Fate!'

All that can be concluded from this brief summary of the responses of a number of adult stutterers is that the range of ideas amongst them is as wide as amongst those who have studied the subject more objectively. It is in many ways very similar to the views expressed by American parents of twenty years ago. Heredity seems, from this sample at least, to be losing its sway, however. Very few adults relate their difficulty to a discrepancy between talking and thinking, as compared with Johnson's parents. And the percentage of 'don't knows' is even higher. It would be interesting to try to discover the effect that these ideas have on the stutterers' attitudes to their problem. We have found that an exchange of these views in a group is one very good way of beginning a dialogue amongst the people who really matter, as to the nature of the disorder they are trying to cope with.

It will be seen from this chapter that there is very little in the way of 'hard fact' about stuttering for any of us to go on. It is small wonder that stutterers, their families and friends and the interested public at large have little satisfaction when they come to the 'experts' for information and help. Before we move on to the developmental aspects of the disorder in the following chapter, however, and discuss the manifestations of disfluency brought together under the label 'stuttering', let us end this section with what 'facts' there are. Though 'the incidence and prevalence of stuttering may show variation from one culture to another' (Beech and Fransella 1968, 28), it is generally accepted that in this country and the USA about 1 per cent of the population are persistent, as against transitory, stutterers. Stuttering almost always begins in early childhood and is at least three times more common in males than in females. There is 'no obvious relationship between IQ level and stuttering' (Beech and Fransella 1968, 28), and socioeconomic factors are unlikely to be of any significance.

6

Developmental aspects of stuttering

The development of fluency in children

Stuttering almost always begins in early childhood, and in many cases disfluency, whether it be called 'normal nonfluency' or 'stuttering', is preceded by a period when speech is fluent. Andrews and Harris (1964) found, for instance, that only 21 per cent of the 80 children studied were said to have been disfluent since the onset of speech. Just over 35 per cent had had 'some fluent speech' prior to the onset of disfluency in the pre-school period, over 28 per cent had 'speech well established' and began to stutter in the infant school, while 14 per cent had 'a long period of fluent speech' and no trouble until junior school. Many parents report that their children have spoken 'quite normally' and stutterers themselves remember having no difficulty. It would seem pertinent, therefore, to consider the development of fluency in children, before we see how this comes to be disturbed by the nonfluencies typical of many children, whether they develop into stutterers or not.

From our study of fluency in earlier chapters it will be seen that this aspect of speech is dependent on the integrated development of many factors. Transition smoothness between speech segments involves articulatory proficiency in the movement from sound to sound and syllable to syllable. A wider linguistic competence will govern the transition between phrases and clauses, with the complex interrelation of semantic and syntactic information and the prosodic features of intonation and stress. Regulation of tempo and pausing have been shown to relate to physiological and psychological factors as well as linguistic context. The natural rhythmical patterns in speech have been discussed, both stress-timed and syllable-timed.

There are many descriptions of the development of spoken language in children and, while their authors may differ profoundly in the way in which they approach the subject, the progressions they outline, from the physiologically based grunts, cries and gasps of the early days to the adult-like utterances of the five-year-old, are remarkably similar. We propose in this section to study this progression briefly, to see how the normal fluency of developed speech is achieved. It should be emphasized at this point that, although the order of the stages of development to be described has been found to be similar in children, whatever language is spoken in their environment, the rate of progression and the extent of each stage will vary greatly. The timing of stages, then, can only be approximate.

The crying and gurgling of the first few weeks can be said to be a part of expressive language only in the sense that the child's state of comfort or discomfort is conveyed to the listener. There is at first no control over or shaping of these sounds, and while they may indicate the presence of a healthy vocal and articulatory mechanism, skill does not yet enter in. Menyuk (1971) has discussed studies of early utterances and notes the evidence of increasing control of the vocal mechanism during the third and sixth month to be found in changes in fundamental frequency of the child's utterances and increased uniformity in their duration. Some authors, including Menyuk (1971, 58), have even made a distinction between the earliest 'unconditioned reflex crying' and 'motivated crying' of this period.

By six months the stage of 'babbling' has begun, when the child 'vocalizes tunefully, using single and double syllables' (Sheridan 1968, 5). There seems to be a good deal of disagreement as to the role of babbling in the child's acquisition of language. Rees (1972) discusses two major theoretical approaches. That of learning theory sees babbling as having an important role in the development of phonological skills and therefore of expressive language as a whole. Those favouring the 'maturational approach' see it as unrelated to later specific articulatory skills. Menyuk (1971, 88) notes an increase in the variety of speech sounds produced in babbling and compares the first articulations, which appear to be 'accidents brought about by chance approximations of the articulators', with later articulations 'brought about by purposeful manipulations of the articulators, by means of which the infant can replicate previous productions'. She relates this change to development of the auditory feedback mechanism and suggests that the infant may be increasingly monitoring his speech productions and testing possible productions. Pitch-change, too, is becoming more varied. The characteristic repetitions of syllables in babbling have often been described as 'vocal play', and it is interesting to remember that Stein (1953) saw the stutterer's repetitions as regression to babbling.

From six to eight months, both adult-like intonation patterns in babbling and imitation of adult intonation patterns have been observed and the period of 'jargon' is beginning. This is described by Menyuk as the phase 'during which children produce strings of utterances marked by intonation and stress, although they produce no clearly identifiable morphemes' (4). Some observers have noted a marked decrease in vocalization following this highly vocal period and preceding the production of 'words'. These early words are neither true adult words nor approximate versions of them, but are distinguished as such when the same speech sound sequence is consistently used by the child in response to a particular object or situation. At the same time, he shows an increasing understanding of speech in his ability to follow simple instructions.

At some point during the second year of life, the child begins to use single, recognizable words which 'vary in prosodic features in a way that makes some sound declarative, some interrogative, some emphatic' (Brown 1973, 153). Clearly there is real meaning here for both speaker and listener and, as Brown points out, 'single words . . . can be expressive of semantic intentions of greater complexity than the naming of referents' (154). They are sometimes referred to as 'single-word sentences'. Similarly, when two-word combinations appear from about two years they often carry the meaning of a much fuller sentence. This meaning is partly conveyed by the child's use of intonation and stress, partly dependent on the listener's knowledge of context. The phonological aspect of the child's speech at this stage shows only approximation to adult pronunciation. Smith (1974) shows how the child reduces the complexity of adult articulation by means of what he calls 'realization rules', such as consonant harmony (i.e. taking an adult word with consonants having different points of articulation and converting it to a form where all the consonants have the same point of articulation). Another is 'cluster reduction' (where two or even three consonants are reduced to one, as in 'tone' for 'stone' (22)).

During the third year of life, the child begins to use longer sentences, often described as 'telegraphic' in nature. These consist mainly of content words (nouns, verbs, adjectives) with many function words (e.g. prepositions, adverbs, conjunctions) omitted. Brown (1973) describes this type of utterance as the reduction of adult language. Word order is preserved in both imitation of the longer sentences of others and in spontaneous speech and, again, intonation and stress are used appropriately to convey meaning. These sentences are intelligible to the listener, just as the telegraphic utterances of some dysphasic adults are intelligible. A difference, however, may be heard in the speed of utterance of the children, who, normally fluent, show no undue hesitations between words, while the dysphasic adults may move in a much more laboured way from one word to the next.

The period between two and four years sees the most evident flowering of phonological and syntactic development in the normal child. The facts about phonological development have been recently summarized by Ingram (1976). Most of the factors involved in the production of adult fluent speech are mastered during this period. By four, the transition smoothness dependent on articulatory facility and linguistic awareness is firmly established. Regulation of tempo, rhythm and pausing is close to the adult model. The basic functions of the intonation and stress systems have been incorporated appropriately for some time (Crystal 1975, ch. 8). The vowel/consonant inventory is well advanced (Fry 1966). Several areas of learning remain, however, e.g. the use of the more subtle structuring and attitudinal functions of intonation (Cruttenden 1974), and the discrimination of certain consonants, especially the front fricatives /s/, /f/, /θ/ (Edwards 1974, Sheridan 1968), which means that the completion of the language's phonological system is not displayed until the child is as old as nine or ten.

In grammar, likewise, the bulk of the learning takes place between 2 and 4 (Crystal, Fletcher and Garman 1976). From the telegraphic, two-element utterances of around two years, the simple (i.e. single-clause) sentence structure develops, until by three, the basic subject–verb–object–adverbial constructions in the clause are well established in a range of different functions (e.g. statement, question, command). At around 3, more complex sentence structure comes to be introduced, using coordinating and subordinating devices, and the main grammatical systems (such as the pronoun, tense and modal system) develop rapidly. The various inflectional endings of words are also firmly established by 4. By this stage, then, most children in their spontaneous speech give the impression of having completed the learning of the grammar of their language (e.g. Gesell 1954, Menyuk 1972).

There are, however, several further developments which must take place to achieve identity with the adult grammatical system, such as the learning of sentence-connecting features, more complex variations in word order, or the distinguishing in comprehension of apparently similar sentences (Chomsky 1969). These further developments occupy children at least until puberty, at which point the learning of grammar seems, to all intents and purposes, complete.

These chronological norms are at best averages based on the research in language acquisition, which on the whole has investigated only middle-class children. They also disregard the known differences between girls and boys (the former's linguistic learning progressing more rapidly than the latter's), and such distinctions as that between fast and slow learners within each category (Ramer 1976). No mention is made here of norms of development in children's awareness of the *use* of these structures, a point which has attracted the attention of the mother-tongue education literature (see the review in Crystal 1976) as well as the language acquisition literature (e.g. Sachs and Devin 1976). But the main outline of structural development *per se* should be enough to provide a perspective for establishing a relative order of events in the emergence of nonfluent linguistic behaviour. If we take 4–5 years as the period when 'language is now essentially complete in structure and form' (Gesell 1954, 53), then it is very evident that many children have become disfluent before this time. As far as we know, no child has ever been reported as being nonfluent up to the appearance of true words. Babbling and jargon, it appears, always remain undisrupted. Some children show hesitations and repetitions (to be described in more detail in our next section) from the time they begin to use single words. (In the study referred to at the beginning of this chapter, Andrews and Harris 1954, it was the more severe stutterers who showed this early onset.) Many more children have begun to use sentences before disfluency occurs. (Johnson, for example, found only three who had not in his 1955 study.) A further group become proficient speakers, only to begin to have difficulty in the next few years. A high percentage from each of these groups experience only transitory disfluency, as we shall see.

It is tempting to see the ever-increasing demands on linguistic competence and articulatory proficiency as a major factor in the onset of some disfluency. Both Andrews and Harris (1964) and Morley (1957) find some evidence of a tendency for speech to be delayed in stutterers and for these children to show a higher incidence of articulatory defect and to attain intelligibility later than non-stutterers. Since by far the greatest number of stutterers are first diagnosed as such between the ages of three and five-and-a-half years (boys) and three and five years (girls) it would seem that the most vulnerable time coincides with just that period when a much fuller use of connected speech is developing.

Bloodstein (1974, 392) suggests that 'It hardly seems far fetched to ask whether some children during this time are so sensitized by the difficulties they encounter in learning adult syntax that, especially if they are subject as well to communicative pressures, they tend to acquire the feelings that express themselves in tense and fragmented realizations of the grammatical structures of language.' But since, as we have said, a large number of children begin to stutter after language has developed normally and fluently, a linguistic factor can only be seen as a possible link with onset in some cases of disfluency and many of these remit as language and articulation reach proficiency. For example, only one of the 37 children studied by Morley remained a persistent stutterer and two had 'a residual and very occasional minor degree of hesitation at times of stress'. All of the children were said to have achieved normal language by five years and to have no defects of articulation by six-and-a-half years. At a later stage of well-established stuttering, there can be no doubt that any difficulty in the use of language or in articulation exacerbates the fluency problem and has probably been closely linked with it from the beginning.

The development of disfluency in children

It will be clear from our discussion of theories of stuttering in chapter 4, that there is considerable disagreement about what is 'normal' in the way of nonfluency in speech and what is 'abnormal'. Some authorities make a neat distinction between the word and phrase repetitions of normal nonfluency and the additional sound and part-word repetitions of children destined to be stutterers. Andrews and Harris (1964) concur with this distinction from their review of studies. The word and phrase repetitions have been said to occur without effort and apparently without awareness on the part of non-stuttering children. Van Riper (1954, 352) sees this as the child's 'hesitancy in completing his thought', while the sound and part-word repetitions seem to him to represent a 'difficulty in uttering his words'. Bloodstein (1970), however, while agreeing that 'stuttering' children produce many more sound and part-word repetitions, found that the speech of non-stuttering children was not free from such disfluency and, in addition, contained the sound prolongations and even evidence of forcing said to belong only to stuttering. As mentioned in chapter 5, he also found evidence of the consistency effect in the speech of normally fluent children, suggesting that they, too, anticipated trouble on certain words to some extent. For Bloodstein and others, then, there is no clear distinction between the characteristics of normal nonfluency and early stuttering symptoms, except as a matter of degree.

Another cause of confusion lies in the concept of 'primary stuttering', a term first used by Bluemel (1932) to describe disfluent behaviour without the fears and associated motor symptoms of the more developed disorder. As long ago as 1953 Glasner and Vermilyea became disturbed by the looseness with which this term was used by therapists and questioned 171 clinicians as to their understanding of its meaning. As they feared, replies were wide ranging. Some saw the term as an alternative word for normal nonfluency, others used it to describe greater disfluency but 'without awareness', and still others allowed of some awareness, but said that the child showed no 'secondary symptoms' (presumably of facial contortions, associated movements or avoidance). As Bloodstein points out (1970, 30), 'We now have a situation in which it would be quite possible for a given set of observations on the same child to lead to a diagnosis of "stuttering" by one professional worker, of "primary stuttering" by another and of "normal nonfluency" by a third.' He advocates an approach to early disfluency which avoids this confusion by simply identifying 'several describable forms of childhood speech interruption' and tracing their development 'without allowing ourselves to become unduly disturbed about the question of how to categorize them' (31). This we propose to do, in asking ourselves in what manner young children are disfluent, and in what contexts, both linguistic and situational.

Bloodstein produced his three papers on the development of stuttering in 1960 and.1961, before he began work on his continuity hypothesis, so that we should perhaps understand his references to young stutterers as now meaning children showing a degree of disfluency beyond that of those regarded as non-stutterers. He traces development in four phases (1960b): *phase 1* representing his observations of mainly preschool children, but the characteristics of which may persist until age seven or later. The first point he makes about this early phase is that disfluency is usually episodic. Fluent periods are very common, and even as these become shorter and less frequent, disfluency shows much wider fluctuation than it will, if it continues, in later years. Disruption tends to occur on the initial word of the sentence to a far greater degree than in more advanced phases and there is a marked tendency for it to occur on function words, especially prepositions, conjunctions and pronouns (the last two being found typical of normal-speaking young children too, on later investigation (Helmreich and Bloodstein 1973)). By 1974 Bloodstein was linking these points of loci of disruption in his hypothesis that the child's disfluency represents fragmentation of whole syntactic structures, in contrast to the older stutterer's fragmentation of words.

Although the most characteristic symptom of early disfluency is, as we have said, repetition, especially of syllables and monosyllabic words, hard contacts or blocks are also quite common. Where they occur on plosive or 'stop' sounds they may produce hard repetitions of the initial sound of the word or complete 'blocks', while on continuant sounds a prolongation results. Associated symptoms of facial grimace, body movements, gasping and speaking on ingoing breath may also be present at this early stage. These disruptions occur most frequently when the child is under some sort of 'communicative pressure'—when he is excited or telling a long story. Yet although there may be brief emotional reactions to severe difficulty, these are usually transitory and there is 'essentially no fear or embarrassment'. The child does not react to himself as a stutterer and 'speaks freely in all situations'.

Bloodstein points out the extreme variability of symptoms of disfluency in the young child and notes the wide range of severity and frequency with which they are manifested. Yet in even some of the most marked cases, disfluency does not persist and the child may pass through this phase and experience no further difficulty. Young (1975b) has questioned the available data for recovery from stuttering, which is not surprising in view of the difficulties of deciding what the use of the term really represents. But it does seem clear that spontaneous remission is common in young children up to the age of 6 or 7 years. The studies of Andrews and Harris (1974), Morley (1957) and Johnson (1959) bear this out.

From here we propose to refer more confidently to 'stuttering' in discussing childhood disfluency, since after this, in its persistence and the beginnings of a self-concept as a stutterer, it does have the attributes of 'disorder' in relation to communication for the speaker as well as the listener. Bloodstein sees *phase 2* as having a number of characteristics which distinguish it from phase one. First, 'the disorder is essentially chronic'. While there may be fluctuations in occurrence and severity, 'it may no longer be said to come in discrete episodes' (370). Secondly, there is a marked increase in stuttering when the child is hurried or excited. The third point concerns the loci of stuttering. Now the disfluency occurs primarily on content words rather than function words, and not so frequently at the beginnings of sentences as formerly (though this tendency is still present in much advanced stuttering). Lastly, although the child still speaks freely in all situations, he now reacts to himself as a stutterer. Typically, there is little concern about stuttering, however, except in severe cases or moments of unusual difficulty. The author does not attempt to place an approximate age to the end of phase 2 as, for some, it may last into adulthood.

Phase 3 shows an increase in difficulty which becomes more specific to certain situations. Similarly, particular sounds are perceived as 'difficult' and anticipation of them has begun to develop. This brings with it the growth of devices for postponing the attempt on the word by, for example, filled pauses or a repetition of the word or phrase preceding it. 'Release' devices, such as the sharp exhalation of breath to terminate a block or head jerking, are more evident now. Despite this, however, 'there are few deep feelings of fear or embarrassment and essentially no tendency to avoid speaking'. Bloodstein states (372): 'Phase three represents fully developed stuttering without the avoidance of speech.' He sees the outstanding characteristic of this phase as 'the contrast between the stutterer's elaborately developed symptomology, with its devices for postponement, starting and release and the attitude of comfortable equanimity with which he appears to accept practically every opportunity to engage in speech'. The age limits of this phase are very broad and may include children of eight years as well as many adults.

It will be seen that in his discussion of the progressive stages in the development of stuttering, Bloodstein is not concerned with relating particular symptoms or the severity and frequency of their occurrence to his phases, and his links with age are of the loosest. What most clearly distinguishes one phase from the next is the speaker's relationship with the act of speaking. In phase 1 there is essentially no disturbing feeling of abnormality in the child, though there is evidence of some awareness in many. In phase 2 the stutterer sees himself as such, but typically feels little concern. In phase 3 there is more reaction and there may be 'exasperation, annoyance or disgust', but the fear and embarrassment and the avoidance of speech involved in *phase 4* (which we shall discuss in chapter 7) are not part of the stutterer's experience. In the phases we have described so far, then, the effects on communication, both for speaker and listener, will depend far more on the severity and duration of the interruption than on the underlying emotional factors which carry such weight in phase 4.

Van Riper (1971), in his chapter on the development of stuttering, expresses dissatisfaction with the whole concept of stages of stuttering, criticizing not only Bloodstein's phases but his own earlier attempts at categorizing stutterers into Primary, Transitional and Secondary groups (1954). While finding that Bloodstein presents well the enormous range of symptoms to be found at every age level, he is not satisfied with the study on which his data were based because the 418 subjects were investigated over a short span of time. Van Riper sees the need for behaviours to be observed over a long period, so that the development of symptoms in each subject may be studied to show the way in which they change in nature as well as severity. He emphasizes the 'oscillatory' course of development in most stuttering until it reaches its final form. From his own examination of the records of 44 stutterers whom he was able to follow from onset to maturity and many others with whom he had contact for three or four years, he states:

> In most instances, the younger the stutterer, the more he tended to oscillate from one level of severity to another. Periods characterized by many syllabic repetitions on many words alternated with other periods as long as a week or month when only two or three such repetitions occurred per day. Later in development, when frustration reactions with facial contortions and struggle appeared, they would persist for weeks and then give way to the earlier, simpler stuttering pattern. Developmentally, the severity of stuttering seems to see-saw back and forth. (103)

Van Riper therefore proposes 'certain common patterns of progressive change' to replace the concept of phases or stages of development. He uses the case records of 300 stutterers, including the 44 longitudinal studies, as a basis for his four 'tracks' of development, pointing out that 69 of the 300 did not fall into any of the patterns described, and that not all of those who did followed its sequence in every detail. While admitting that his sample may not be sufficiently representative of the stuttering population as a whole, and regretting that only 44 cases were studied at length, Van Riper is sufficiently convinced of the validity of his approach to the progressive development of stuttering to discuss it in some detail. A summary of his findings is contained on the chart on pp. 88-9 (taken from Van Riper 1971, 116-17).

The development described in these four tracks represents changes in behaviour which occur before stuttering is stabilized into its fully developed forms, referred to later by Van Riper as 'advanced' or 'confirmed'. Tracks I and II were by far the most common patterns amongst the cases studied. Those following track I were already showing signs of potentially severe effects on communication in the increase of fear and avoidance. For those on track II, with no signs of withdrawal in the face of their difficulties, the experience of stuttering was much less painful, though their listeners would probably have found the repetitious interruptions, combined with excessive speed, equally disturbing and certainly more confusing. Of the smaller number who followed track III, Van Riper notes that although a good many of them recover at this stage of development, those who do not become very severe stutterers. The symptoms described in the final section of track III show a combination of growing emotional difficulty and increasingly complex and abnormal motor behaviour. Thus the effects on communication are directly experienced by all concerned. Of the few track IV stutterers, Van Riper believes that they 'suffer less than their listeners'. And he sees 'controlling, punishing, wheedling, exploitive urges behind the behaviour' (115).

While Bloodstein's developmental phases show us most clearly the changing relationship towards communication which may occur when (and if) the stutterer passes from one phase to another, the great value of Van Riper's approach would seem to lie in his differentiating between types of progression. In our last chapter, we referred to the agreement between many who have worked on the problem of stuttering that we are dealing with a number of related disorders, rather than a single one. And while Van Riper has not been able to produce a definitive study with the data available to him, this method of observation over time surely contains within it the possibility of clarifying differentiated disorders as they develop and diverge from one another. Sixty-nine is too large a number to be excluded for us to accept the four tracks as representative enough to cover stuttering groups as a whole. Forty-four is too small a number studied from onset to maturity. But a great deal more could be learnt about the nature of different types of stuttering if the time and resources were available to analyse the progress of disfluency patterns in this way. This, together with much more clearly defined data in relation to onset might teach us much of what we need to know in order to provide adequate preventive measures and effective treatment.

Attitudes towards communication and the development of self-concepts in young stutterers

In our consideration so far of the development of stuttering in children, we have mainly been concerned with the physical symptoms related to disfluent behaviour, and have only touched on growth and change in emotional reaction to this disfluency. Any assessment of the disorder (which we will discuss in our next chapter) must take into account the stutterers 'feelings about his speech and his attitude toward interpersonal communication in general' (Erickson 1969, 711). Much attention has been paid to the attitudinal dimension of stuttering, especially in recent years. Most of what has been written, however, refers to 'advanced' stutterers. In this section we will attempt to trace the development of this aspect of the disorder from the growth of awareness of disfluency, up to the stage where the stutterer's view of his world has begun to be dominated by his communication problem.

Our first difficulty, of course, lies in defining our terms. There is disagreement as to what the word 'attitude' implies, as Insko (1967) points out in his introduction to his book on theories of attitude change. Drever (1952, 22) defines an attitude as 'a more or less stable set or disposition of opinion, interest or purpose, involving expectancy of a certain kind of experience and readiness with an appropriate response'. This definition seems to us to hold the necessary elements covering most fully what we understand by the stutterer's attitude towards communication, especially in its implication that a certain response develops as the result of expectancy of a particular kind of experience.

Similarly, the term 'self-concept' appears to have very different implications for different writers, as Van Riper (1971) shows in his chapter on the subject. He restricts his use of the term to 'self-awareness, self-identity and self-evaluation'

At onset

Track I	Track II	Track III	Track IV
Begins 2;6 to 4 years	Often late—at time of first sentence	Any age after the child has consecutive speech	Late; usually after 4 years
Previously fluent	Never very fluent	Previously fluent	Previously fluent
Gradual onset	Gradual onset	Sudden onset, often after trauma	Sudden onset
Cyclic	Steady	Steady	Erratic
Long remissions	No remissions	Few short remissions	No remissions
Good articulation	Poor articulation	Normal articulation	Normal articulation
Normal rate	Fast; spurts	Slow, careful rate	Normal rate
Syllabic repetitions	Gaps, revisions, syllable and word repetitions	Unvoiced prolongations; laryngeal blockings	Unusual behaviours
No tension; unforced	No tension	Much tension	Variable tension
No tremors	No tremors	Tremors	Few tremors
Loci: first words, function words	Loci: first words; long words; scattered throughout sentence; content words	Beginning of utterance after pauses primary	First words; rarely on function words; content words especially
Variable pattern	Variable pattern	Consistent pattern	Consistent pattern
Normal speech is well integrated	Broken speech with hesitation and gaps even when no disfluency	Normal speech is very fluent	Normal speech is very fluent
No awareness	No awareness	Highly aware	Highly aware
No frustration	No frustration	Much frustration	No frustration
No fears; willing to talk	No fears; willing to talk	Fears speaking; situation and word fears	No evidence of fear; willing to talk

Developmental characteristics

Track I	Track II	Track III	Track IV
Repetitions of syllables increase in frequency and speed and become irregular	Behaviours remain the same but the speed increases; their number also increases	An increase in the frequency but the behaviour at first changes little; signs of frustration	The number of instances increases and they are shown in more situations
Then:			
Repetition of syllables begin to end in prolongations	Little change in form	More retrials are seen; lip protrusions and tongue fixations appear; prolongations of initial sounds	Little change in form; monosymptomatic and symbolic
Then:			
Prolongations show increased tension, tremors, struggle; evidence of frustration	Little change; little awareness; little frustration	Tremors; struggling; facial contortions; jaw jerks, gasping; marked frustration	Little change
Then:			
Overflow of tension; facial contortions; retrials; speech output decreases; signs of concern	Duration of nonfluencies increases; more syllabic repetitions; little awareness	Interruptor devices become prominent; rate slows; more hesitancy; more refusals to talk	Little change in type but duration and visibility increase; no interruptors or new forcings; increased output of speech
Then:			
Situation fears join other behaviours and avoidance behaviours; then word fears and fears of certain sounds	Occasional fears of situations, not of words or sounds; long strings of syllabic repetitions	Intense fears of words and sounds; many avoidances; patterns change in form and grow more bizarre; output of speech much overflow; will cease trying to talk. Poor eye contact; normal speech becomes hesitant. Nonvocalized blockings are frequent. Primary tonic* blocks with multiple closures	Very few avoidance or release behaviours. Not much evidence of word fears. Few consistent loci. Very aware of stuttering. Stutters very openly. Good eye contact. Little variability in stuttering behaviour. Normal speech very fluent. Talks a lot. Consistent pattern; few silent blockings. Either tonic* or clonic*

* Van Riper describes the term 'tonic' as referring to fixatory behaviours, while the term 'clonic' refers to oscillatory or repetitive behaviours. It would seem to us less ambiguous to refer to 'blocks' or 'hard contacts', as we have earlier defined them, and 'sound repetitions'.

(200). We, however, propose to take a fuller description, which we find satisfactory. Clark and Murray (1965, 132) define self-concept as 'the mental representation an individual has of his own body or "self". Emotional experiences, fantasies, postural changes and internal sensations, contact with people and objects, successes and failures all unite in forming an individual's self-concept.' Quoting an earlier study by Clark and Fitzpatrick (1962, 164) they continue: 'It includes both the conscious and unconscious attitudes, memories, feelings and fairly stable characteristics that one has regarding himself and his place in society. It is an individual's reaction to his bodily and mental processes.' It will be clear from this description, which includes attitudes as part of the self-concept, that the experience of communication through speech will play a large part in the development of such a concept, wherever there is disorder of any kind. Speech having both physical and psychological attributes, a great deal of the 'self' is involved in the process. And since it is largely a social activity, the reactions of the environment, as well as of the individual, will have a strong influence on the way in which a stutterer's concept of himself develops.

Fransella (1972) writes in terms of 'personal constructs' rather than 'self-concepts', and although her approach has many distinctive features (as we shall see in chapter 7) much of her discussion of the stutterer's 'system of ideas' about himself and his world is relevant to this question of how the child builds up his concept of himself in relation to his disfluency. She doubts whether fluent children 'ever do establish a very elaborated subsystem to do with speech in the normal course of events'. That is, they take speech for granted as they do other abilities such as walking. Disfluent children, however, may come to develop a strong focus of attention on speech, initially through parent–child interaction. A mother, for instance, may become concerned that a child 'stumbles too much in his speech. She may be anxious about it because Uncle Harry stuttered, or she may simply be concerned that he "get it right". Whatever her reason she draws attention to his speech.' Then, 'He begins to discriminate between, say, the sounds he makes to his mother and the sounds he makes when by himself' (65). The emphasis, she points out, is on his disfluencies, not his fluencies. Though there may be no anxiety in the child at this stage, Fransella sees this emphasis as the beginning of a system of ideas about himself that will have implications for him in the future. It is striking in work with adult stutterers that while they so often notice and react to every disfluency, they have the greatest difficulty in registering equally strongly the far higher number of fluencies which almost all of them produce.

From this early drawing of attention to a 'difference' in speech, we can only speculate as to how a child may develop to the stage of 'brief emotional reactions' to the more severe difficulty experienced in moments of excitement in Bloodstein's phase 1. Since fear and embarrassment have been observed to be absent, frustration (the first emotional reaction to be noted by Van Riper in his track I development) is likely to be the child's strongest feeling. This is apparent in young children faced with all manner of difficulties in using growing skills. Furthermore, adults as well as normally fluent children tend to react with frustration to momentary speech failure, through mispronunciation or loss of the appropriate word.

In his description of phase 2, Bloodstein (1960b, 370–4) says that the child 'thinks of and reacts to himself as a stutterer' but has 'little or no concern about his stuttering except in severe cases or at moments of unusual difficulty'. This phase begins, he says, 'as soon as relatively long, fluent intervals cease and the child has acquired a self-concept as a stutterer'. But he does not say how this concept develops from the transitory moments of self-consciousness about speech experienced during the earlier phase. Van Riper (1971, 200) seems to be describing a much later stage of development when he says: 'there is no doubt that the person who says of himself "I am a stutterer" formulates his self-concept in a way that implies compulsive deviancy. . . . As stuttering develops, there comes a time when, as a result of his own communicative frustration and the social rejection he gets from others, the stutterer comes to label himself as such.' It is difficult to see what Bloodstein means by the child's having a 'self-concept' as a stutterer, and Van Riper seems to relate self-identification to a stage of experience far more complex and long-standing and certainly beyond the period during which the child feels 'little or no concern'. Perhaps Bloodstein sees the child as having a concept of himself as a stutterer from the point at which he actually learns to say that he 'stutters'. But, since he is not troubled by the fact at this stage, he can hardly have begun to relate very much of his experience to this particular idea about himself. He may, however, already be beginning to build up an embryonic system of focusing on moments of difficulty and setting them apart from less strongly registered experiences of fluency.

By phase 3, not only are these experiences becoming less frequent but certain situations, words and sounds are perceived and anticipated as giving trouble and are split off from the rest of the child's communication. The postponement and release devices described earlier which surround the utterances serve to highlight them further. Although there is said to be no avoidance of speaking in terms of situations or communication with particular people, earlier occasional frustration may have developed to reactions of 'exasperation, annoyance or disgust'. These latter imply the growth of a more critical attitude towards disfluency as undesirable behaviour than the simpler expression of frustration.

To Johnson (1959), of course, listener reaction and evaluation play a major part in developing the child's attitude towards his communication problem, and children will vary in their experience here. A child with highly critical parents, unsympathetic teachers and mocking school-friends will be far more likely to learn to regard his stuttering with shame and to anticipate difficulty with dread, than another who has been less harshly treated. The second of Johnson's 'major variables', 'the speaker's degree of nonfluency as objectively determined' is clearly also relevant. Where the child's stuttering is frequent and severe, and involves distracting associated symptoms, he will not only experience it himself more vividly, but be subject to more negative reaction. The third variable, 'the speaker's sensitivity to his own non-fluency and to the listener's evaluative reactions to his nonfluency' will also develop to a different degree in children according to the development of their self-concept as a whole.

Although we can see to some extent the gradual changes in attitude which may occur as the child continues to stutter and to experience a wider range of reaction to his disfluency as his environment widens, there is as yet little data to help us discover the extent to which his concept of himself as a whole may be affected by these changes in attitude. It is possible that before the stage is reached where stuttering is a 'way of life' (Fransella 1970) rather than a speech problem, the child stutterer is able to view himself as a speaker separately from the rest of his attributes. (And, as Bloodstein maintains, many stutterers do not develop beyond phase 3 into the situation where almost every experience is governed by the disorder.) One study by Woods (1974, 741) lends some support to this idea.

Forty-eight stuttering boys, whose ages ranged from 8 to 12 years, were compared with 562 of their normally fluent classmates in terms of 'social position' and 'speaking competence'. The primary purpose of the study was to discover whether children as well as adults have predominantly unfavourable expectations concerning the personality characteristics of stutterers. If this is so, Woods felt, 'their evaluations and reactions toward the stuttering child could be a powerful influence in shaping his self-concept'. He attempted to 'obtain the children's evaluations of their stuttering classmates' speaking competence and social position, to assess the stuttering child's awareness of these evaluations and to determine the degree to which speaking competence and social position are related for third-grade and sixth-grade boys who stutter'. The results imply that while both the stutterers themselves and their peers considered the 48 boys 'poor talkers', this did not affect either the fluent boys' ratings of their 'social performance' or the stutterers' expectations of how they would be rated. Some adults do, of course, report adverse reactions from children at school, but most seem to have taken any teasing because of their stuttering as they would being mocked for red hair or some other distinguishing feature.

If, then, the majority of young stutterers, do take their disfluency in their stride, as we suspect from their lack of concern in treatment, what are the factors within themselves and within the environment which change the situation for so many of them? Discussion with adult stutterers has revealed that most of them clearly remember a time when their disfluency did not matter to them too much. Most seem to agree that their earlier memories are of particular bad moments, rather than a more or less constant questioning in the back of the mind as to whether they were going to stutter or how they were going to handle this or that speaking situation. The process of change seems to be part of a much more fundamental change in their approach to life, associated with yet one more ill-defined term—adolescence. Hadfield (1962, 180) suggests that we use this word 'growing-up' of the teenage period alone because we are speaking of the time when 'the youth is leaving behind the phase of protective childhood and is becoming independent, capable of going out to fend for himself'. Most young people at this stage begin to formulate their expectations of themselves and more is expected of them. A greater self-consciousness about abilities, looks, attractiveness and many other aspects of their personalities develops and a greater sensitivity to the attitudes of others towards them. Some of the adult stutterers, attempting to express these changes, relate their growing concern about their speech to social situations—

relationships with members of the opposite sex or meeting more strangers. At the same time, many are beginning to think about future work and the effect that stuttering will have on prospects there. Pressure of examinations is often suggested as a reason for an increase in stuttering. Clashes at home, especially with parents, with the fundamental problem of communicating differences of opinion and desires that these imply, drive some into silence, others into intense arguments.

Even such a brief and superficial glance at this period of development suggests that it is a time when both the speaker and his environment may make greater demands on 'performance' in general and speech in particular. Going back to Clark and Murray's definition of 'self-concept', we can see how many aspects will be affected by the individual's experience of speaking. Increasing consciousness of 'bodily processes' and concern about appearances will make the physical dimension of stuttering more vivid. 'Contact with people' and growing concern about 'his place in society' will make the evaluations of others matter far more, and the effects of others' judgements about his abilities and personality will relate more directly both to his idea of himself now and his evaluation of his potential for the future. If 'successes and failures' do indeed play a part in the development of the self-concept, speech failures must be registered high among them. It is small wonder, then, that the awareness of disfluency often changes to 'expectancy' of stuttering and 'readiness with an appropriate response' either of stuttering itself or a whole pattern of behaviour to avoid stuttering. Nor is it surprising, with speech playing such a major part in all our lives, that many stutterers begin at this stage to relate more and more of their experience to the single fact that they stutter.

The treatment of stuttering in children

Although the scope of this book does not allow for discussion of treatment methods in depth, we cannot leave this chapter on the developmental aspects of stuttering without a brief survey of therapeutic approaches with children. Clearly, these will depend to a large extent on the standpoint of the clinicians concerned as to the nature and cause of the disorder. Weinstock (1968, 17) discusses the dichotomy which he believes exists in therapy for stutterers in the public school system in America. Speech therapy, it appears, is ranged on one side, focusing directly on the stutterer's speech and seeking 'amelioration of stuttering behaviour'. Psychiatry opposes this speech-focused approach, feeling that 'stuttering is a symptom of a more fundamental emotional conflict, originating in early formative experiences'. Moreover, 'until the symptom need is resolved, hitting at the symptom or drawing attention to it only makes the patient cling more tenaciously to it'. Against this claim, the speech clinicians are said to feel that they cannot really call any more attention to the stuttering than already exists, that these symptoms can themselves be the cause of 'personality distortion', that, in fact, 'the "symptomatology" is the disease'.

Although these two extremes of view can be found both in America and this country, treatment procedures for stuttering in children and adults can be seen to fall into much subtler gradations from one to the other, with the majority of approaches combining concern both for the psychological aspects of stuttering and the disfluency itself. With children, treatment is viewed developmentally and the approach changes according to the stage a particular child has reached. The most comprehensive discussion of therapy for very young children can be found in Van Riper (1973, 372). He calls his chapter 'Treatment of the beginning stutterer: prevention', which is perhaps the one linking aim in all the approaches, from whatever point of view. From his review of American and British literature he finds two main points of agreement for this level: that 'the stuttering itself should never be worked on directly' and that 'one of the basic goals of therapy is to reduce the communicative stress felt by the child'. In general, 'therapy' is carried out at home by the parents, under the guidance of the clinician. They are asked to inhibit their own reactions to the child's disfluency, to protect him from interruption and too much competition, remove any time pressure when he is trying to tell something and prevent 'emotionally disruptive influences' and excitement as far as possible.

In Europe, however, Van Riper finds that there is much more direct fluency training, with work on all kinds of rhythmic activities and attention to language development as a whole. In many clinics, especially in the Iron Curtain countries, very young children are treated directly and intensively in residential groups, away from their families. This is in complete contrast to the view expressed by Brook (1957, 32) and held by many therapists in the West that 'A child who attends a speech clinic regularly is likely to discover at an early date that he suffers from stammering and this step is to be avoided where possible.'

Despite the basic points of agreement in the West as far as treatment of the young child's disfluency is concerned, approaches to the psychological aspects of stuttering vary widely. Those who view the disorder in terms of neurosis or early conflict may work with the child himself, through play therapy, or attempt to resolve the conflict through the parents. Some clinicians advocate psychoanalysis for the parents, especially the mother, others hold less formal interviews with them, where they may express their anxieties about their child and discuss means of preventing the development of the disorder. Van Riper points out that simply handing out 'advice' to parents will do more harm than good. In his experience, most parents 'have not been highly disturbed or maladjusted individuals . . . but they did need some chance to complain and explain and wonder and wish. They needed someone to share their hopes and fears and troubles before they could change their management of the stuttering child or alter the environment in which he had to exist and communicate.'

Van Riper's own approach to the beginning stutterer, while less rigorous than some Europeans, is far less passive than many therapists. He sums up what he believes a 'skilled clinician' can do as follows:

(1) He can make the child's speaking pleasant again
(2) He can stimulate the child with models of fluency that are within the child's reach, models which, when imitated, will increase the child's own fluency
(3) He can provide activities that integrate and facilitate the smooth flow of utterance

(4) He can programme schedules of rewards and reinforcements for fluency that will enhance it

(5) He can desensitize the child to those stimulus conditions which tend to disrupt his fluency

(6) He can countercondition other anxiety inhibiting responses to the same fluency disruptors

(7) He can prevent the moments of stuttering from acquiring the stimulus value which so often leads to avoidance and struggle. (399)

In conclusion, Van Riper feels that, 'with all these opportunities to ameliorate the problem, it seems unwise to delegate all the responsibility to the parents. Therapists are trained to do these things; parents are not.'

With older children, fully aware of their speech difficulty, many of the treatment procedures followed with adults are used, with suitable adaptations, and we shall discuss these in our next chapter. But two main differences should be mentioned. As we have said, the majority of young stutterers do not experience the fear and embarrassment suffered by many adults. And while this in itself is an advantage, it can bring with it lack of motivation either to concern themselves with the nature of their disfluency or to work to control it. Secondly, it is far more difficult for the young person to perceive exactly what the disrupting behaviour is and to change that behaviour when asked to do so. Demonstration of an alternative way of saying a 'hard' word is more appropriate at this level than description of a technique.

Briefly, therapy with the young 'confirmed' stutterer has as its main aim the prevention of the development of adverse emotional reactions to disfluency and the avoidance of speech which so often goes with them. The child is encouraged to enter all normal speaking situations, given specific practice with particular difficulties and as much opportunity to experience his fluency as possible. Group work is on the increase and appears to provide 'a potentially more interesting and stimulating environment for the child' (Fawcus 1970) than much individual therapy, at this stage of his development. Once again, it is Van Riper (1973, ch. 15) who provides us with both the most comprehensive survey of treatment for these older children and the most practical suggestions from his own work at this level.

Recovery from stuttering in children

In an earlier part of this chapter we emphasized the problems involved in the diagnosis of stuttering in young children. Data concerning onset is ill-defined and the exact nature of early disfluency disputed. No discussion of recovery from stuttering, therefore, can hope to reach any firm conclusion. Where figures are based on the reports of the 'recovered stutterers' themselves, as in Sheehan and Martyn (1970) and Cooper (1972), we find estimates as high as 80 per cent. Young (1975b) disputes such findings, however, criticizing them as 'verbal reports of past events', rather than 'direct observation'. Andrews and Harris (1964) give a similar percentage of recovery for the 43 children identified in their survey as stutterers.

Young points out, however, that the disfluency experienced by many of the children was of such short duration that we should question their ever having 'stuttered' at all. He further emphasizes that the term 'stuttering' is even more loosely used amongst laymen than clinicians, so that replies to questionnaires from either the young people themselves or their parents about earlier stuttering are suspect. Also, views as to what counts as recovery vary. All we can say with any certainty is that a high percentage of preschool children recover from periods of disfluency before they are five years old. Thereafter, the recovery rate decreases, although it can occur at any stage in the development of the disorder. While some adolescents experience an increase in both the severity of symptoms and emotional reactions, others re-acquire fluency at this stage (see Wingate 1964). As we shall see, however, recovery in the young and older adult becomes rarer as the demands on communication increase.

7

Stuttering in adults

It will be seen from our discussion of stuttering in children that the disorder does not simply progress from easy, repetitive disfluency to more severe and more complex speech interruptions. Not only may hard blocks and gross associated movements be found in quite young children, but many adults remain free from such symptoms. A child of eight years may delay 'difficult' words by intrusion of inappropriate sounds or release fixed articulatory postures with a violent jerk of the head, while an adult may never have developed such features. Although the characteristics ascribed by Bloodstein to his phase 4 are 'more typical in older adolescence and adulthood', all of its features may be found in a child as young as ten years of age and some of them even earlier. We are not, then, concerned in this chapter only with the severest forms of stuttering or with those whose experience of their speech problem is thus outlined by Bloodstein (1960b, 374):

(*1*)   vivid anticipations of stuttering
(*2*)   special difficulty in response to various sounds, words, situations and listeners
(*3*)   frequent word substitutions and circumlocution
(*4*)   avoidance of certain speaking situations
(*5*)   other evidences of fear and embarrassment

Our justification for separating the adult stutterer from the child relates much more to differences in communicative responsibility and in effects on communication for both the adult speakers and their listeners.

One term we can use in relation to the widely differing patterns of disfluency which we shall be discussing is Van Riper's 'confirmed stuttering' (1971). Whatever the fluctuations in severity and despite the occurrence of periods of fluency for some at this stage, the pattern is now set. A particular speaker will not always manifest every symptom in his repertoire when he stutters, but, with a few exceptions, some of them the result of therapy, these do not change over time except in degree. Successful therapy will, of course, eliminate some or even all of them, as will a change in circumstances. On the whole, however, where no attempt is made to change the pattern it remains stable.

Overt manifestations

In our previous chapter we have already mentioned many of the possible overt symptoms to be found in adult stuttering, including some of the associated body movements. The literature abounds in lurid descriptions (e.g. Van Riper 1971, ch. 6) and we do not wish to add to the drama surrounding the disorder with more. We propose, however, in this section to examine some of the most common overt stuttering behaviours, both in terms of the involvement of the speech mechanism and their effects on the utterance as a whole. At the same time, it seems important to distinguish those disfluencies which are also to be found less frequently in the speech of non-stutterers from others which are characteristic only of stutterers.

Although inappropriately timed and located contacts may be observed at any place of articulation, many believe that the stutterer's primary difficulty lies in the onset of phonation. Wingate (1969a), for example, sees the initiation of phonation as 'a crucial element in the complex of stuttering' and maintains that it is the constant need for transition from voiceless to voiced sounds which makes reading and conversation so much more vulnerable to disfluency than, say, whispering, which entails no phonation. In a second paper (1969b) he describes stuttering as 'a phonetic transition defect'.

In a study of the physiological and aerodynamic aspects of fluency and stuttering, referred to in chapter 3, Adams (1974, 37) describes fluency as dependent at least in part 'upon the correct timing and the prompt smooth initiation and maintenance of air flow and glottal vibration'. These effects are said to result from 'the harmonious integration of subglottic pressure, glottal resistance and supraglottic pressure'. Any activities which cause the disintegration of these variables prevent the timing, starting and maintenance of air flow and concomitant vocalization. He feels, therefore, that those muscle actions might well be the motor determinants of stuttering. He gives an example of how such disruptive action could destroy fluency (38):

> Suppose, in attempting to start talking, an individual experiences simultaneously a drop in subglottic pressure and an abnormal rise in glottal resistance. As long as these disturbances were extant, they would seriously reduce the speaker's chances of immediately meeting the need for air flow and phonation. The overt manifestation of this particular disintegration might be a prolonged silence, possibly accompanied by a fixation of the articulatory posture needed for the first phoneme in the first word to be uttered.

In an earlier paper Adams and Reis (1971) tested their hypothesis 'that the frequency with which vocalization must be initiated in a given speech segment and the frequency of attendant disfluency are positively related'. A group of 14 stutterers were given two passages to read five times, one containing all voiced sounds and the other mixed voiced and voiceless. The latter entailed more 'off-on' phonatory adjustments than the former. Statistical analyses all showed that there was significantly less stuttering and more rapid adaptation associated with the all-voiced material. They conclude that 'at least some of the universally demonstrable characteristics of stuttering (that is, repetitions and prolongations) demonstrated by many of the subjects in this study reflected the difficulty these individuals had initiating or maintaining phonation and co-ordinating it with articulation so as to make fluent transitions from sound to sound and syllable to syllable'. Young (1975a) criticizes the mode of analysis in this study and doubts whether the results really do support the hypothesis. While acknowledging some of the points Young makes with regard to adaptation, Adams and Reis (1975) do not concede their basic position. It seems likely that the debate, which, as Young points out, began in the early part of this century, will continue well into the next.

Although it may be arguable that all repetitions and prolongations are produced because of difficulty in initiating voice, a number of disruptions may occur which probably have their origin in the larynx and in the subglottal region. The silent blocks referred to by Adams (1974) which often entail breath-holding and 'freezing' of all activity, are perhaps the most striking and can cause considerable discomfort in the listener. Exhalation of breath before an utterance, without phonation, may also occur as well as intrusion of inappropriate laryngeal sound, for example 'vocal fry', as described by Van Riper (1971, 135), a sharp 'hiccoughing' sound, voiced inhalation, as well as very frequent filled pauses, typical to a lesser degree of many non-stutterers. Some stutterers make hard attacks on vowels, producing vowel repetitions. The repetition of a consonant may be regarded either as a failure to initiate the following vowel or as the result of a hard attack on the consonant itself. To the speaker and the listener, the sound repeated or prolonged seems to be perceived as the difficult one, whether this be so or not.

The plosives /p, b, t, d, k, g/ are in many cases approached with such a tense closure of the articulators that sound only emerges in a violent burst after a pause, during which the speaker can be seen trying to force it out. Here again, the long stoppage at, say, the lips for /b/ may be seen as secondary to a failure of phonation or as the primary block. We believe, with Van Riper (1973, 133) that it may be one or the other in different instances. Sometimes the articulatory closure for a plosive is actually accompanied by laryngeal sound, so that we hear as well as see the struggle behaviour. (See Appendix for some of these features.)

Some investigations have been made into the particular sounds which stutterers experience as 'difficult'. Johnson and Brown (1935) reported a great variation amongst individual stutterers, but found more instances of stuttering on initial consonants than on initial vowels of words. Soderberg (1962) discussed phonetic influences upon stuttering and compared vowels, voiced consonants and voiceless consonants. He attempted to equate his word lists in terms of frequency of word usage in the English language, readability, word length, position of words in a phrase, accent of initial syllables of words, and grammatical function of words. He found no evidence of differences among vowels, voiced consonants and voiceless consonants with respect to the mean frequency of stuttering instances or mean duration of stuttering instances, thus disagreeing with previous studies.

In a later paper (1966) Soderberg considered the relationship of stuttering to word length and word frequency. His results agreed with other studies in finding a significantly greater frequency of stuttering to be associated with increases in word length and decreases of word frequency. Word length, he found, was the more potent of the two variables in its effect on the frequency of stuttering. Wingate (1967) also studied the question of stuttering and word length and found it to be an important variable associated with stuttering and independent of both grammatical class and phonetic difficulty. In a much earlier investigation, Brown (1938, 119) had considered stuttering in relation to word accent and word position. His conclusions were that stuttering occurs more frequently on accented than unaccented syllables in the majority of cases and that 'the objective data bear out stutterers' introspections concerning the psychological primacy of the beginning of the word'. Finding that accented syllables and the first words of sentences were more frequently stuttered, he suggested that increased activity of the speech mechanism and the relatively greater tension required at these points might be a possible explanation. He also felt that the stutterer's desire to avoid stuttering at these crucial points might also be a factor in the occurrence of disfluency.

In a later paper (1945), Brown considered the loci of stuttering in the speech sequence and found that the first three words of sentences elicited stuttering more often than the remaining words and that this was independent of phonetic and grammatical factors. He also found, as have others, that longer words tended to be stuttered more than shorter words. Grammatical classes found to elicit more stuttering were adjectives, nouns, adverbs and verbs, while pronouns, conjunctions, prepositions and articles gave less trouble. He concludes (605):

> It is probably in terms of the evaluation of words as being conspicuous, prominent or meaningful that the loci of stutterings are to be accounted for. . . . The significance of such evaluation of a word by the stutterer appears to lie in the fact that having so evaluated a word, he desires to avoid stuttering on it. He reacts accordingly with caution, hesitancy, effort, conflict etc. and it is predominantly those reactions which are termed stuttering, as contrasted with 'normal' or non-stuttered speech interruptions.

Brown himself admits that his study is neither 'elegant' nor 'definitive', but his conclusions seem to be sound.

The blocks described earlier are only one of the ways in which stuttering may manifest itself. It may be remembered that many have considered sound repetitions in young children to be one of the distinguishing features of stuttered speech, as against normal nonfluencies. Prolongations of sound occur in the speech of those considered fluent, but far less frequently, and hard contacts are rare in normal speech. Fluency also involves smooth transition between larger segments than phonemes, however: between syllables, words and phrases. Repetitions of syllables, words and phrases may also be marked disruptors in the speech of stutterers of all ages. Here, with phonation itself so actively involved, it is difficult to see its onset as the core of the problem. (For a summary of these features, see Fig. 5, p. 48.)

Syllable or 'part-word' repetitions have been found to be stuttering character-istics, though by no means unknown amongst fluent speakers, while word and phrase repetitions are common to both, but more frequently heard from those who stutter. Syllable repetitions tend to occur in normal speech when the speaker has difficulty in pronouncing a polysyllabic or unfamiliar word. Word and phrase repetitions are often used by fluent speakers as an alternative to pausing, when a particular word is being sought. They serve the same function as interjections of other words and phrases. Although these same 'normal' nonfluencies may occur in the speech of stutterers, they also occur in the face of a sound or word associated through past experience with a block, where there is no doubt as to the pronunciation of a word and they know all too well exactly the word they wish to say.

In some severe forms of stuttering, not only syllable repetitions but sound repetitions, prolongations and hard contacts may occur in the middle of a word as well as initially. These disruptions can be very confusing for the listener, causing them to ask for a repetition of the utterance, which invariably leads to more stuttering. It is the more severe stutterers, too, who may insert additional inappropriate sounds at the beginnings, ends or in the middle of words, sometimes rendering them unintelligible. Difficulty over initial sounds may occasionally be dealt with by omitting them altogether or articulating them silently. Perhaps the most extreme example we have heard of a disturbed articulatory pattern consisted of initial sound repetitions, followed by a vowel, with the rest of the word unspoken. Since prosody, too, is severely disrupted in such a case, meaning is almost entirely lost. Generally speaking, stress and intonation are retained in more moderate degrees of stuttering of all kinds. With severe forms of the disorder, output may show reduction of these features or, in a few cases, appropriate intonation is retained to a remarkable extent, even over a very slow and laboured utterance. This seems to provide possible additional evidence for the idea, discussed in chapter 2, of the tone-group as the essential unit of neurolinguistic programming.

Breathing abnormalities, such as gasping, speaking on residual air or on inhalation, the forcing out of breath before a word is attempted, are common to many types of stuttered speech. Some stutterers present for treatment complaining that their breathing is the cause of their difficulty. In our experience, however, these abnormalities most often are the result of stuttering, not the cause. It is seldom necessary to do direct work on breathing, as this becomes normal as other aspects of disfluency subside. There is a tendency in some, however, to go on talking without renewal of air when they are speaking fluently. This seems to indicate a real fear of stopping the flow with any kind of normal pausing, in case they are unable to start again. Here it will be necessary to pay direct attention to phrasing and the proper use of breath.

We have already touched on some of the inappropriate body postures to be found, and there is a wide range of them, together with tongue protrusion, facial grimaces, eye-closures or eye-fixation, head-jerks and jaw-jerks. Most of these may be seen as release devices. It is believed by many therapists that at some stage a jerk of the head, click of the tongue or particular eye-movement has been successful in releasing a block, then become part of the stuttering 'ritual'. Similarly, hand and arm, leg and even trunk movements develop in some stutterers as part of the struggle to produce utterance. It is the bizarre nature of some of these behaviours which causes embarrassment and even fear in many listeners. It is almost impossible for someone unfamiliar with such symptoms not to be completely distracted by the grosser physical manifestations. Some stutterers are not aware of many of them. One man recently saw himself on a videotaped recording, producing severe facial contortions, heard himself grinding his teeth and realized that, due to frequent very fast repetitions, he was extremely difficult to understand. Fortunately, he is a determined man and the experience simply increased his motivation to inhibit such behaviour, which he proceeded systematically to do.

Sheehan (1974, 193) summarizes details of overt stuttering behaviours from a phonetic analysis made some years before of 500 stutterings; 25 were taken from 20 adult stutterers and his findings are as follows:

(1)   Repetition and prolongation were the only behaviours common to all.

(2)   The average duration of 1·6 sec., with a standard deviation of ·3 sec.

(3)   The mean length of the prolongations was 0·87 sec., with a standard deviation of 0·72 sec.

(4)   More than 4 out of 5 repetitions (83 per cent) were phoneme and syllable repetitions.

(5)   Phrase repetition was comparatively rare, amounting to only 5 per cent of the repetitions.

(6)   There was a strong tendency for various stuttering behaviours to be aligned into a definite sequence or stuttering pattern.

(7)   Ninety-six per cent of the stuttering occurred in relation to initial sounds.

(8)   One-half of the blocks involved some degree of stuttering on the wrong sound.

(9)   Stutterers frequently continued to stutter on words they had already said.

(10) Stutterers described as their 'hard' sounds the initial sounds they actually uttered successfully, to the exclusion of the remainder of the word.

(11) Stuttering was seen chiefly as a disorder of release, with irrelevances and crutches employed as instrumental acts to satisfy fear and bring about the termination of the block.

It is to be hoped that we have made it clear that adult stutterers vary greatly in the type and number of overt symptoms they produce, as well as the frequency with which these disrupt their speech. Some may, for instance, produce only repetitions, some only blocks in moments of disfluency. Others may show most of the kinds of interruption described in the course of an utterance of any length. We have mentioned that even 'confirmed' stutterers may have their periods of fluency or only occasional difficulty, and all of them show increases and decreases in severity according to a number of criteria: particular speech situations, certain listeners, the size of the group in which they are speaking among them. It is generally assumed that an increase in disfluency automatically indicates an increase in the anxiety experienced by the speaker. Although this is often the case, as it is with some non-stutterers, there are other factors to be taken into account. Some stutterers for example, stutter more, not less, with family and friends, with whom they feel relaxed. When they achieve a degree of control through therapy, they are surprised to find that it is more difficult to exercise it in familiar surroundings than new ones. This suggests that for them at least, association plays a stronger part in perpetuating disfluency than anxiety. Although each individual has his own 'list' of situations in which he is typically more disfluent, examples such as telephoning, buying tickets, shopping, stopping a stranger in the street, speaking to someone in authority, rank high for many of them. Many stutterers can be completely fluent when alone and experience some of their greatest difficulty when meeting strangers for the first time. Many react to excitement, time pressure and the tension and fast speaking of others with an increase in stuttering. Fatigue generally has an adverse effect on fluency, but anger can work either way. Role-playing or assuming an unaccustomed voice or dialect often produces, at least temporarily, greater fluency, as has been found with our clients at the City Literary Institute.

Psychological aspects

Although we found in our discussion of theories as to the nature and causes of stuttering that there is little to suggest that the disorder is itself emotionally based, our attempt to trace its development through childhood revealed, in many cases, a clear growth of covert reactions, which we will now consider in relation to stuttering in adults. We saw how awareness of difficulty may develop into reactions of frustration and the beginnings of fear and avoidance. Some of the overt behaviours already discussed themselves indicate anticipation of and attempts to deal with a 'dangerous' word: the delaying tactics, the release mechanisms. Loss of eye-contact as trouble looms is a common reaction of many stutterers and this can generalize into an almost total inability to look at the listener when speaking. As Argyle has shown (1975), eye-contact is a very important aspect of personal interaction. Van Riper (1971, 166) sees the 'intense scanning of a prospective utterance' as one of the most prominent features of the confirmed stutterer, an exaggeration of the in-process monitoring discussed in chapter 2. Some are so skilled in this that they seldom stutter, managing to substitute one word after another for those on which they anticipate disfluency. Circumlocution is a common method of word avoidance, sometimes producing a fluent utterance of great length in place of a brief statement, sometimes leading to confusion and even more stuttering. Other devices range from pretending to forget a particular word to remaining silent when an intended statement contains a potential stutter.

The decision not to speak can have far-reaching effects when it is made continually in the face of speaking situations as a whole. Always shopping in a supermarket, instead of asking for things over the counter, using ticket machines instead of asking for a destination, may in themselves be simply minor inconveniences. But deep frustration and shame can result from habitually remaining silent in conversations where the person feels he really has something to say, or persistently failing to make those initial verbal contacts which are a part of establishing human relationships. Some stutterers avoid going to places where their speech difficulty might be exposed to strangers and even choose jobs entailing the minimum of speech. Although it should be emphasized that many people, even with severe speech problems, do not become isolated and withdrawn through communication fears, some undoubtedly feel that stuttering has restricted their lives greatly, with respect to work and social life, and to a large extent hindered the development of their personality as a whole.

There are many factors governing the stutterer's ability to tolerate speech failure. Some of these must lie within the person concerned and relate to a more general resilience and capacity to bear frustration. His concept of himself as a whole, partly dependent on his experience of the reactions of others, will make the fact of stuttering the one area of dissatisfaction with himself or only part of a more total sense of inadequacy. Some stutterers are acutely aware of each moment of disfluency, while others remain undisturbed by knowledge of even quite bizarre behaviour. For these and many other reasons, on which we can only speculate, the stutterer's view of the severity of his problem may not be directly related to the severity of overt symptoms.

One important point is relevant here. People, including many speech therapists, are often puzzled by the apparent ease with which some quite severe stutterers, never free from their difficulty for any length of time, seem to manage to live with their problem, while others, who have little observable trouble, express far more concern and experience much more intense situation fears. There is a tendency to assume that the former are particularly 'well-adjusted' people, while the latter must have some basic psychological vulnerability, be essentially 'over-sensitive' and lacking in courage. But while both assumptions may be quite true in some cases, it should be realized that a speaker who stutters consistently and inevitably is experiencing something quite different from another who is fluent a great deal of the time, but who knows that he may suddenly be caught in a moment of stuttering which will shock his listeners as well as himself. It must in some ways be easier to accept inevitable disfluency, to which listeners also become accustomed, than the constant threat of possible disruption. More consistent stutterers are also relieved of any conflict between being open about their difficulty and trying to hide it.

But undoubtedly, however well a speaker may deal with the fact or the fear of stuttering, by the time he has reached adulthood his speech probelm must consist of more than the surface manifestations of abnormal sound and movement. The relationship between overt and covert aspects is not clearcut. Joseph Sheehan (1970, 15) expresses the disorder in terms of an iceberg, with the statutory nine-tenths beneath the surface, consisting of 'concealment behaviour, false roles, tricks, fear, avoidance, guilt, shame' and the far smaller proportion above of the 'stuttering behaviour' itself. Neat as this analogy may be, it seems clear that there is wide variation amongst stutterers in the proportion of 'hidden' as against 'open' behaviour. They also differ greatly in their ability to observe and express the covert aspects of the problem, just as some are more able than others to appreciate the nature of the overt symptoms. In fact, as has often been pointed out, there are probably more differences to be found between stutterers themselves than there are between the two broad groups of stutterers and fluent speakers.

Assessment

With so wide a range of overt symptoms to evaluate, and covert reactions to take into account, the assessment of stuttering is extremely complex. We saw how subjective ratings of early disfluencies prove to be, and although there is less controversy over the existence of most confirmed stutters, there are still difficulties in obtaining objective measures of both the nature and severity of the disorder in its later forms. As far as the disfluencies themselves are concerned, we have not only to decide *what* we are going to assess but *when* we should assess, since their occurrence is so variable for most speakers. How, too, can we make an adequate evaluation of the covert aspects of stuttering, when they may be 'hidden' not only from us, but from the speakers themselves? How important is the stutterer's own evaluation of the severity of his problem which, we have suggested, to some extent governs the effect of his stuttering on his listeners as well as himself? We clearly must have as full and careful an assessment as possible, not only as a tool for analysing every aspect of a particular form of the disorder, but as a means of judging the effects of any attempt to ameliorate it.

Perhaps the most comprehensive attempt to assess stuttering in depth is that of Johnson, Darley and Spriesterbach (1963). They set out to study significant aspects of the speech behaviour itself, the speaker's own reactions to stuttering and the reactions and attitudes of listeners. For the first of these, a classification of eight types of disfluency is used (pp. 209–10):

(*1*) interjections of sounds, syllables, words, phrases
(*2*) part-word repetitions
(*3*) word repetitions
(*4*) phrase repetitions
(*5*) revisions (e.g. where the pronunciation of a word or the content of a phrase is modified as in 'I was—I am going')
(*6*) incomplete phrases (where the thought or content is not completed)
(*7*) broken words (e.g. 'I was g- [pause] -oing home')
(*8*) prolonged sounds.

The stutterer is asked to complete two speaking tasks: the 'job task', speaking for three minutes about present or future job, and the 'TAT' task, where a card from the Thematic Apperception Test is presented and he is asked to tell a story based on the picture, also taking three minutes. In addition, a reading passage containing 300 words is used. Taperecordings of all three are analysed, the disfluencies categorized and counted. Measures are taken of the number of disfluent words per minute in the speaking task as well as the rate of speech (i.e. the number of words spoken in three minutes) and, for the reading, the number of disfluencies and rate of speech or time taken to complete the 300 words.

As a detailed account of the speech behaviour of a stutterer at the time of testing, this is very thorough. Johnson and his colleagues add to this a long check-list, including types of disordered breathing, abnormal articulatory postures, eye-closures and movements of the head and body to be specified by an observer (279). The severity of stuttering is then rated on a seven-point scale, from '(*1*) Very mild—stuttering on less than 1 per cent of words; very little relevant tension; disfluencies generally less than one second in duration; patterns of disfluency simple; no apparent associated movements of body, arms, legs or head' through to '(*7*) Very severe—stuttering on more than 25 per cent of words; very conspicuous tension; disfluencies average more than four seconds in duration; very conspicuous distracting sounds and facial grimaces; very conspicuous distracting movements.' Andrews and Harris (1964) and others have pointed out that such a scale is probably too detailed for general clinical use, 'for not only is it difficult to use with reliability, but a significant proportion of stutterers will vary between groups from day to day' (4). They themselves suggest a much simpler grading from 0 to 3:

Grade 0   stutter not heard at interview
Grade 1   mild stutter; communication unimpaired; 0–5 per cent words stuttered
Grade 2   moderate stutter; communication slightly impaired; 6–20 per cent of words stuttered
Grade 3   severe stutter; communication definitely impaired; over 20 per cent words stuttered

They reduce Johnson's eight categories of disfluency to three: simple repetitions; prolongations and hard blockings; associated facial and body movements.

Andrews and Ingham (1971) also found that rate of speech correlates highly with the severity of stuttering and consider that speech which is free of stuttering but below the normal rate (140±24 words per minute) still sounds abnormal. Therefore they present the percentage of words stuttered together with the number of words spoken per minute as a good indication of the extent of communication impairment.

We agree that the seven-point scale of Johnson *et al.* is both cumbersome and too specific in its detail to be reliable. (Where, for instance, would we place the stutterer who has more than 25 per cent disfluency, but the average lasting only two seconds and few conspicuous movements?) But reducing the categories of disfluency to just the three suggested by Andrews and Harris or doing away with them altogether, as in simple counts of 'disfluent' words, seems to us to lose a great deal of necessary detail. Although all classifications are inevitably to some extent arbitrary, to say that someone with 19 per cent words stuttered is only a moderate stutterer, with communication slightly impaired, while one who stutters on 20 per cent of words spoken is severe, with communication definitely impaired, is not very satisfactory. The listener's perception of the severity of stuttering is, of course, in part dependent on frequency of occurrence, but, as we have suggested, the nature of the disruption in both its audible and visible aspects would seem to be of great importance in terms of its effects on communication. Nor do percentages of improvement in terms of reduction of disfluencies and time saved fully convey the subtler changes from, say, a very tense, struggling pattern to one that is more relaxed, within the speaker's control, and thus allowing for greater freedom of communication. Perhaps the use of a seven-point scale for percentage of disfluencies without the details of behaviour stipulated, plus a brief description of the individual's types of disfluency, movements etc. together with the time taken, would give the clearest rating and allow for more detailed comparison with reassessments than the Andrews and Harris.

More difficult than the question of *what* to assess, however, is that of *when*. It is likely that in an initial assessment most stutterers will produce their severest level of disfluency in the clinic. Something more is needed, though, to pinpoint the variations in severity which occur in other situations in their daily lives. Short of following each stutterer with hidden camera and microphone for about a week, we must rely on his subjective self-rating for information. Usually, each person is presented with a list of situations related to his work or college life and social environment and asked to rate himself in terms of the severity of the stuttering he would expect. Johnson *et al.* ask for more than this in their 'Stutterer's Self-Ratings for Reactions to Speech Situations' (288). They want to discover (*a*) the degree of avoidance on a 5-point scale, from 'I never try to avoid' to 'Every time I possibly can', (*b*) reactions, from enjoyment to intense dislike of a situation, (*c*) stuttering, from 'very rarely' to 'severely', and (*d*) frequency of meeting a situation, from 'very often' to 'rarely'.

With 40 situations to consider from these four points of view, this is a long task. But is has the merit of showing us several dimensions of the problem from the speaker's point of view. Responses to (*a*) should give a very full picture of the degree of avoidance generally practised. (*b*) tells us something of the stutterer's attitude towards communication as a whole, and (*c*) his estimation of the seriousness of his disorder. (*d*) is important in that the degree of involvement in speaking situations may have a bearing on the isolation or otherwise of a particular stutterer from communication with others. The situations covered are very much oriented to college life and, it seems, specifically American college life. It should be possible, however, for the content of the questionnaire to be suitably adapted to the lifestyle of those attending adult clinics in Britain and elsewhere.

The main objections to both clinical ratings of disfluency and self-ratings seems to lie in retesting to evaluate the effects of therapy. Andrews and Ingham (1972, 300) remark: 'A longstanding suspicion of many clinicians is that "successfully" treated stutterers can often produce fluent speech for a formal or overt assessment.' This is especially true when the therapist who has worked with them is the assessor. They suggest, therefore, that a better measure of sustained improvement would be 'extended interviews, during which the subject is oblivious to a covert assessment of his speech'. In their study, the subjects were interviewed by undergraduates in their own homes, under the impression that they were taking part in a project related to the undergraduates' psychology course. In a later paper, Ingham (1975) discussed the results of reassessment of a group of stutterers some time after treatment. It was discovered that with retesting at three months after a course, the percentage of stuttering showed a significant increase in recordings of which they were unaware but at six months, such a difference between the two conditions was no longer found. In our experience, the awareness of a speech evaluation date does signal a time to increase vigilance over their speech for most stutterers coming for periodic review and, on the whole, has the effect of producing greater control of disfluency. This suggests, as some have stated, that there is therapeutic value in the very fact of being 'followed up', since the increased vigilance does not only apply to the period of actual testing. Since follow-up studies should be for the benefit of the stutterer as well as the clinician in evaluating progress, perhaps a combination of the two types of retesting would be useful.

As far as the validity of self-rating is concerned, the difficulty here is that the speaker's evaluation of the severity of any stuttering episode may change in the direction of leniency with a positive change of attitude or become more critical, where growing control of disfluency produces higher aims. One way of counteracting the latter, which we have found useful, is to let the stutterers hear an earlier recording of themselves, as a reminder of just what their disfluency behaviour has been in the past. They often forget former aspects of their stuttering which they have overcome. Since, however, self-ratings are, by definition, subjective and have their main value in expressing the stutterer's impression of the seriousness of his problem, perhaps they should simply be left alone and judged primarily in those terms and only secondarily as additional measures of how he is actually performing outside the clinic.

Assessing communication attitudes

Since the stutterer's attitudes towards communication in relation to his speech difficulty are so important a part of the disorder, it is clear that an effective measure of them is as necessary to our assessment as the evaluation of disfluency itself. Erickson (1969, 711) claims that up until that time 'little systematic investigation of stutterers' attitudes toward their own or other's communication behaviour had been reported'. Various attempts have been made to measure attitudes towards stuttering itself, as in the Iowa Scale (Ammons and Johnson 1944), but, as Erickson points out, data have not been published to demonstrate the validity of measures obtained and the scale tends now to be used more as a guide for clinical interviewing and counselling than as a standardized assessment tool. Woolf (1967), in his Perception of Stuttering Inventory (PSI), tried to go deeper than the purely behavioural measures of the severity of the problem by asking the speaker to evaluate his disfluent behaviour in terms of 'struggle, avoidance and expectancy'. While it does reflect the stutterer's attitudes towards his stuttering and provide a useful means of helping him to understand his overt behaviours, it cannot, as Andrews and Cutler (1974) stress, be used to determine general communication attitudes and any changes which may occur through treatment.

Erickson (1969), on the assumption that stutterers would differ from non-stutterers in their attitudes towards verbal communication, devised his S-scale (see p. 96) of 39 items relating to a wide range of speaking situations. He found (and Andrews and Cutler (1974) have supported his findings) that responses to the S-scale were a valid index of the extent to which the stutterers' attitudes towards communication deviate from the norm. One hundred and twenty stutterers and 144 non-stutterers completed the scale, and while both groups showed a wide variation of responses, the stutterers' scores ranged from 6 to 37, with a mean range of 25·65, while those of non-stutterers ranged from 2 to 33, with a mean of 13·24. Since stuttering or any other speech disorder are not the only sources of communication difficulty, we should expect some overlapping, but the scores of 95 per cent of the stutterers were higher than the median score of non-stutterers. Andrews and Cutler (1974, 315), wishing to adapt the S-scale as a tool for retesting, i.e. to determine changes in original attitudes through treatment, reduced the items to 24, selected out of the 39 'because they discriminated between stutterers and non-stutterers, showed a strong trend toward normalcy when administered to stutterers improving in treatment and proved reliable when repeatedly administered to non-stutterers'.

Erickson's 39-item S-scale

The items deleted in the adaptation by Andrews and Cutler (1974) are in italics. The remaining items constitute the S24 scale. Asterisks indicate the response scored positively.

I usually feel that I am making a favorable impression when I talk	True	False*
It is easy for me to talk to important people	True	False*
More than anything else I would like to be able to talk better	*True	False
You can't gain much by arguing	*True	False
I find it easy to talk with almost anyone	True	False*
I find it very easy to look at my audience while speaking to a group	True	False*
I have felt self-conscious when reciting in class	*True	False
A person who is my teacher or my boss is hard to talk to	*True	False
I am often in places where I need to introduce one person to another	True	False*
I would like to introduce the speaker at a meeting	True	False*
I never did volunteer much to recite in class	*True	False
Even the idea of giving a talk in public makes me afraid	*True	False
Some words are harder than others for me to say	*True	False
I would rather not introduce myself to a stranger	*True	False
I forget all about myself shortly after I begin to give a speech	True	False*
I am a good mixer	True	False*
People sometimes seem uncomfortable when I am talking to them	*True	False
I dislike introducing one person to another	*True	False
I often ask questions in group discussions	True	False*
I find it easy to keep control of my voice when speaking	True	False*
I become suddenly afraid when called upon to speak	*True	False
I do not mind speaking before a group	True	False*
I find it easiest to talk with persons younger than me	*True	False
I do not talk well enough to do the kind of work I'd really like to do	*True	False
My speaking voice is rather pleasant and easy to listen to	True	False*
I am sometimes embarrassed by the way I talk	*True	False
I face most speaking situations with complete confidence	True	False*
There are few people I can talk with easily	*True	False
I talk better than I write	True	False*
My speech is the same as always	True	False*
I wish it did not bother me to talk with people	*True	False
It is easier to answer questions in class than to ask them	*True	False
I often feel nervous while talking	*True	False
In school I found it very hard to talk before the class	*True	False
I find it hard to make talk when I meet new people	*True	False
I often have to search for the words I want	*True	False
I feel pretty confident about my speaking ability	True	False*
I wish that I could say things as clearly as others do	*True	False
Even though I knew the right answer I have often failed to give it because I was afraid to speak out	*True	False

Score: _____

Andrews and Cutler believe that in their revised S24 scale they have produced an instrument which adds 'a new dimension of information about the pathology of the condition that is not accounted for by measuring the frequency of symptoms' (316). Although research at the City Literary Institute is only now in progress, using the scale as part of the assessment battery, a glance at the results of responses by twenty of the adult stutterers coming for intensive therapy during the past year seems to suggest that they can indeed be used diagnostically. In several cases, where a stutterer with a mild level of disfluency (below 5 per cent) scored high on the S24 (above 20), the emphasis in treatment needed for them proved to be much more on their anxieties about stuttering than on techniques for control of the symptoms. One or two with low scores on the S24, but severe disfluency (over 20 per cent), responded more readily to the techniques and showed less interest, because of less need, in discussions on attitudes and situation fears. While these different therapeutic needs would emerge during the course of treatment, such indications given right at the beginning would allow for more appropriate initial planning in the balance of behavioural and psychological aspects of therapy offered to particular individuals or subgroups within the context of intensive group work.

The effects of stuttering on communication for the speaker

We have suggested throughout these chapters on stuttering that the disfluency itself, and the speaker's attitude towards that disfluency, will have widely varying effects on communication for different people. For some at least, almost total withdrawal may result, affecting the development of abilities in the work situation and both the maturing of relationships within the family and the establishment of new ones in the wider environment of a normal social life. For others, of course, stuttering does not have this severely limiting effect on personal interaction. But for most 'confirmed' adult stutterers the fact of stuttering will make communication with others a distinctly differing experience from that of normally fluent speakers in a number of ways. Although many jobs do not depend heavily on the ability to express oneself effectively, all those entailing a large number of exchanges either with colleagues or members of the public will be far more difficult or even impossible for a stutterer to carry out. The play situations of childhood are largely replaced for the adult in his social life by talk. Any involvement in local affairs or wider national issues demands a great deal of speech. The bringing up of a family is bound to be hindered by any serious limitation in verbal communication.

We have asked a number of adult stutterers attending speech therapy courses at the City Literary Institute to outline the ways in which they feel communication is affected for them, and certain points recur. Perhaps the main one expressed is the sheer absorption they have in their speech problem, whether it be mild or severe. Though by no means all of them experience deep anxiety a great deal of the time, most of them are on the alert for trouble, scanning their next utterance for prospective disfluency. Some of them felt that this made them poor listeners, unable to attend fully to what was being said to them. Many of them, particularly the more severe stutterers, also spoke of the amount of energy, physical and mental, taken up by stuttering or endeavouring not to stutter. Some are exhausted by the effort after speaking for any length of time. One actually came for treatment principally because of this exhaustion, another was about to give up his work as a general practitioner, because the effort of talking to forty or fifty patients in a day left him with no energy for any family or social life.

All felt that, to some degree, their options as communicators were narrowed. Not only were certain activities accessible to fluent speakers considered out of their reach, such as taking part in committees, debating societies, drama groups, even spontaneous discussion in a larger social group, but what they did say was limited in many ways. Several spoke of cutting down any explanation needed to the bare minimum, simplifying an argument to the points they felt they could make easily. Some gave up argument altogether, agreeing with another speaker rather than getting involved in complicated disagreement. Others even spoke of saying the opposite of what they felt, because it happened to be easier, or producing speech full of contradictions, as they floundered through avoidances. One of the aims of therapy must be to open out these options, in part through increased fluency and in part through reconceptualizing the roles into which they have become settled as a result of their disfluency.

For those who do not opt out of speech when they anticipate difficulty, the effect of disfluency on thought and language can be very disturbing. Failure to say a word can produce a 'blank' in the mind as to what the original idea was they were trying to express. Avoidance of words can lead to total confusion or, at best, inappropriate expression, which puzzles the listener as well as the speaker. One man gave the example of intending to ask who was to be in charge of a group of people on a gliding expedition. He actually said: 'Who is the executive head?' and he remembers to this day the blank stares he met in response. The therapists were under the impression for several weeks that a member of a group was engaged to be married, because, when asked if he was married he replied, 'Pending'. What he meant to say was that he was divorced, but he was having great trouble with 'd' at that time. Quite a common delaying device which can render speech almost unintelligible is the use of interjectory phrases until the desired word 'comes through'. One example consisted of: 'in point of fact, by and large, to put it another way, how shall I express it . . .' until the speaker himself had forgotten what he was trying to say. Some stutterers become very skilled at 'talking about nothing', which in fact is a more total form of avoidance. The results can be amusing, but they are seldom informative or very satisfying to the speaker himself.

Many who do opt out of expressing themselves verbally find that, when they achieve greater fluency, their lack of experience makes it extremely difficult to marshal their thoughts into speech. They never have tried to explain a point, describe an event or express their feelings in words, and these things require practice. Though their use of words and syntactic structure in writing may be perfectly adequate, they may have trouble not only with vocabulary, but with syntax in more complex speech. These people, too, may be very tentative about the pronunciation of words which they have never actually uttered. A verbal skill such as telling a joke effectively also needs practice, and several spoke of the frustration of not feeling able to tell one when a situation seemed to cry out for it. As well as being unable to be witty, they have often failed to be either complimentary or critical when they wished. Several of them felt that they had adopted a somewhat passive, conciliatory role which was false to them. Some overcompensate at times of greater fluency and talk for the sake of talking, unable to handle the normal give-and-take of real conversation. (They should be reassured, however, that many so-called 'normal' speakers share this problem.)

These are just a few of the ways in which communication with others may be affected in some degree for the majority of adult stutterers. Some of them are obvious to the listeners and, in turn, may evoke an embarrassed or at least confused reaction. Others affect only the speakers themselves. A number expressed themselves as being fairly resigned to a limited experience of one of the most important aspects of our lives, but the majority felt, from time to time at least, deep frustration and a very real sense of deprivation.

The effects of stuttering on communication for the listener

We have already indicated in earlier chapters the importance of listeners in stuttering behaviour. We have discussed their role in the early diagnosis and in the development of the disorder and touched briefly on the importance to the stutterer of the reactions of listeners to their speech as he experiences them. As one aim of therapy must be to help the speaker to gain a realistic view of just what these reactions are, studies on this aspect of disfluency are clearly of great importance. They are, however, so far rather sparse, their findings conflicting and mostly confined to investigating reactions to specific types of disfluency, rather than to stuttering patterns as a whole. In this section we will attempt to relate some of the evidence concerning listeners' perception of disfluency as abnormal (that is, 'stuttering'), negative reactions to disfluency, and listeners' concepts about various personality attributes of stutterers.

Several studies suggest that some types of disfluency are more readily judged as stuttering than others. Williams and Kent (1958), for example, found that syllable repetitions and sound prolongations were more often described as stuttering than revisions. Boehmler (1958) showed that sound or syllable repetitions were more often classified as stuttering by observers than any other kind. Sander (1963) found, as we should expect, that double-unit repetitions were more noticeable than single-unit repetitions. Frequency of occurrence must clearly be a factor in the listener's overall judgement of the speaker as a stutterer. Miller and Hewgill (1964) and Sereno and Hawkins (1967) found that six disfluencies every hundred words produced such judgements.

Although there is general agreement as to the types of disfluency classified as stuttering, investigations into the negative reactions by listeners to these different types show conflicting results. Miller and Hewgill (1964) studied the effects of repetitions and interjections on listeners' opinions of the speakers' credibility. Repetitions, they found, produced more negative effects than did interjections. Duffy, Hunt and Giolas (1975), however, found that of broken words, part-word repetitions, prolongations and interjections, the last produced more negative reaction. These authors studied the effects of the four types in terms of listener ratings of 'speaker competence, trustworthiness [i.e. honesty], dynamism and delivery, using semantic differential scales and ratings of attitude toward the topic' (109). Also, they proposed that the amount of information transmitted with each message could be determined by a test of recall of information. With the exception of the more adverse reactions to interjections on some dimensions, mentioned above, there were essentially no differences in ratings of messages containing the four different types of disfluency. All four were rated significantly lower than a fluent reading on speaker competence, dynamism and delivery. On the speakers' trustworthiness, the listeners' attitude to the topic or their recall of the content of the message, however, the differences were not significant. The authors conclude that 'disfluency does not affect the information transmitted in a verbal message, but it can negatively influence the listener's evaluation of the style of delivery and the competence of the speaker'.

An interesting extension of this study would be one in which the frequency of disfluency was much higher than the six instances per 100 words, as it is our impression that severe stuttering (20 per cent and above) *would* be found to affect the information transmitted in a verbal message. All these studies are concerned only with the audible aspects of stuttering. Similar investigations might usefully be made into the effects of combined visible and audible manifestations since this, in many cases, is what the listener experiences in the course of everyday communication with those who stutter.

Fransella (1968) approaches the question of listener evaluation of stutterers from the point of view of their stereotyped concepts of them as a distinct group, rather than their reactions to different aspects of the disorder. She found that fluent speakers tended to see stutterers in rather unfavourable terms. (See also Woods and Williams 1976.) Using a supplied set of concepts which were rated on the Speech Correction Semantic Differential (Smith 1962), she found that the concept 'stutterers' evoked such associations as painful, severe, difficult and tense and that these seemed to link with ideas of guilt, sensitivity and the need to belong. Interestingly enough, stutterers were found to have the same ideas about other stutterers as those held by fluent speakers and yet to have quite different concepts about themselves as individuals. It appears, therefore, that a stutterer generally exempts himself from this unfavourable view, despite his absorption in the fact that he stutters. It seems likely, too, that this exemption will begin to apply to a particular stutterer as the listener gets to know him for more than his speech behaviour and thus to move away from the stereotyped concepts.

There is no doubt that the listener does adapt to stuttered speech. Rosenberg and Curtis (1954) noted that the initial loss of eye-contact in a group of listeners to stuttered speech gradually became less as the experiment went on. As long ago as 1939 Ainsworth studied the breathing patterns of listeners to stuttered speech and found that the disturbance caused early on in the experiment subsided. Anyone working with stutterers knows the dangers of subjectively rating decreases in the severity of disfluency, since the speech therapist undoubtedly adapts even more quickly to disruption than less experienced listeners. These facts probably have implications for the acceptability of the more severe forms of stuttering in a particular job. Where the speaker is communicating with the same people all the time, not only is it likely to be easier for him, but his colleagues will adapt. Where a severe stutterer has to approach new people every day, his listeners do not have this opportunity of adaptation and the effects of his disfluency are likely to be more disturbing. Similar factors apply to the stutterer's social life. A good deal more work would need to be done, however, before such implications could be turned to practical use in terms of guidance.

Treatment

We do not propose in this section to attempt a comprehensive survey of the many different types of treatment for stuttering. In his book devoted to the subject, Van Riper (1973) outlines both historical and current approaches in some detail. We shall be referring to fuller accounts of some of the therapies, as we discuss various aspects of treatment which seem to us to be significant in our understanding of the nature of the problem with which we are trying to deal. We have maintained all along, with other writers, that we are not only faced with a number of different problems, all called 'stuttering', but that with each form of it, especially in confirmed stutterers, a number of aspects must be taken into account when planning treatment. Unfortunately, none of the attempts to classify disfluent speakers into distinct groups have resulted in any useful implications for treatment. And probably they never will. Speakers placed in one group, according to etiological factors, for instance, will not, by adulthood at least, all be producing the same overt symptoms. Nor will they be matched in terms of reaction and attitudes towards communication. The motivation needed for the sheer hard work involved in overcoming most forms of disfluency may be present or absent in particular people, regardless of the type or severity of the disorder as a whole. All therapeutic approaches have their successes and their failures. Some stutterers have 'tried everything' and everything has failed. Others, we suspect, who have succeeded through one method might have succeeded equally well through another.

From so confused a picture it must be clear that a thorough assessment of all aspects of the disorder in the form presented by each client is essential. Only this will guide the clinician in planning the appropriate treatment in broad terms. Where it is found, for instance, at one end of the scale, that the stutterer's speech problem is secondary to a deeper disturbance of personality development, then psychotherapy, such as that outlined by Barbara (1962) or even a psychoanalytic approach (Glauber 1958) may be the most relevant type of treatment. Wolpe (1969) sets out to 'decondition' the emotional factor, where 'neurotic anxiety' is the determinant of stuttering. For the majority, however, their disfluency is not an expression of neurosis, though there may in some be great anxiety in reaction to communication difficulties. For these, the emphasis in treatment must be principally on the psychological aspects of fear and avoidance, but they will need some means of modifying their speech behaviour as well as their emotional behaviour. For others, while anxiety and discomfort play their part in the disorder—and treatment should always encompass them—direct work on the disfluency itself and adjustment to the changes which result from greater fluency must take a prominent position in therapy plans.

Briefly, attempts to modify the speech patterns of stutterers fall into three categories: those which seek to replace stuttering by an alternative pattern of speaking, those which aim at reducing the stutter to an easier, more relaxed form, and those which attempt to eliminate disfluencies by inhibition of disruptive elements. All of these in some way imply reduction of the tension involved in moments of stuttering, whether they take the form of hard blocks, repetitions, associated movements or any of the other behaviours outlined earlier. Relaxation exercises alone have not proved very successful, but relaxation directly related to modification attempts seems to be essential. In general, these techniques are learnt and applied in stages—first with material inside the clinic, where the content of speech does not demand too much thought, such as reading, description of a picture, simple question and answer, then in more creative speech and in communication situations as they occur in life outside. (See Ryan and Van Kirk 1974.)

One of the most commonly used forms of alternative speech patterns practised in this country is syllable-timed speech (Brandon and Harris 1967). Here the stutterer is asked to time his speech to a regular and (initially) slow beat on each syllable that he utters. It is, for most speakers, easily acquired 'because it is essentially a simple mechanical process, utilizing previous language skills' (68), and, being distinct from the normal rhythms of speech, it lacks 'previous learned association with stuttering'. The main objection to the use of syllable-timed speech lies in its abnormality. Although some stutterers are willing and able to use it to good effect outside the clinic, others find it impossible, either because the distracting factors involved in communication prevent them from remembering to apply it, or because they feel it frankly unacceptable to their listeners and themselves. We see its usefulness, not in terms of an alternative to stuttered speech, but as a means of controlling it for some. It may, initially, be the speaker's first experience of having fluency at his command. Having established control in this way, partly through reduction of tension and partly through the slowing-down inevitable with its use, some stutterers can then go on to apply direct modification of symptoms with greater ease. Those who use it skilfully learn to switch into the rhythm to take them through anticipated difficulty and then discard it as they are confident of more direct control. Few stutterers in our experience have continued to use syllable-timed speech consistently, though many have found it useful at an early stage of treatment.

Another approach involving the imposing of an alternative speech pattern at least initially over stuttering is that of 'prolonged speech'. This method was evolved out of experiments with DAF discussed in chapter 5. It was found that many stutterers were fluent under this condition, their speech becoming slow, with each sound drawn out. Goldiamond (1965) worked intensively with DAF apparatus, while Ryan and Van Kirk (1974) dispensed with the apparatus after the initial sessions and the subjects went on to simulate the pattern evoked by

DAF. The advantage of prolonged speech over syllable-timed is that the speaker has only, gradually, to speed up and shorten the prolongations to achieve a normal pattern, while syllable-timed speech, though it may be speeded up and enhanced by normal intonation, will always remain distinct from normal. Recent experiments at the City Literary Institute in London have shown promising short-term results. Using a carefully structured programme of work, beginning at 30 words a minute and moving to 60, then 90 words a minute, with gradual reduction in the length of prolongation, stutterers presenting a wide variety of disfluent patterns have achieved a high degree of fluency in the clinical situation and on outside assignments during the courses. It is too soon to say whether this method also enables them to maintain fluency more effectively and overcome the problem of 'relapse' so common after apparently successful therapy.

Approaches which aim to replace more intense stuttering by a still disfluent but more relaxed pattern have taken many different forms. 'Bouncing', the deliberate repetition of the sound potentially blocked, is one which some stutterers seem to find easier and more acceptable than an imposed speech pattern. 'Pull-out' involves 'dissipating the built-up pressure and making second or even third attempts to utter the blocked sound' (Berlin and Berlin 1964). These authors found that the latter was, on the whole, more acceptable to listeners than the former. The purpose of 'easy-stammering' (Irwin 1972) 'is to learn to replace all stammers with "stammers" without tension. If the first syllable of a stammered word is drawn out sufficiently, it is usually possible to say it without tension' (152). All these methods share the same preference for controlled stuttering over 'artificial' fluency. For some stutterers at least, it would appear that such an approach is more realistic. It certainly implies a gradualness of change which seems essential for many.

The most ambitious form of control is usually referred to simply as 'modification'. Although its final aim is effortless control, as described by Van Riper (1973, ch. 12, 301 ff), it is put into practice in a number of stages. Before any attempt is made to modify, both the overt and covert aspects of disfluency must be identified in great detail. 'Desensitization', aimed at the 'reduction of negative emotion', follows and only then is modification of the disfluency attempted. Preparation for control is provided through the use of masking and DAF for 'the enhancement of proprioceptive monitoring'. 'Cancellation' is the first step—the stutterer is asked to stop after a stuttered word and say it again, the purpose being 'a preventative of stuttering self-reinforcement'. 'Pull-outs', as described earlier, are then attempted as stuttering occurs. By this stage the stutterer is producing a 'new slow-motion form of fluent stuttering' and at the final stage, involving the use of 'motor-planning and preparatory sets', he is anticipating a potential disfluency and meeting it 'in a more normal fashion, integrating the timing of air-flow and phonation and working slowly through the motoric sequence'. This, in effect, replaces the old stuttered pattern by a 'slowed version of the standard utterance'. In many clinics in the UK, a somewhat simplified form of modification is practised, omitting the masking and DAF, cancellation and pull-outs. After a thorough identification, the stutterer is asked to use his anticipation of disfluency to stop, release the growing tension, then attempt the word with a 'light contact' in place of the hard attack habitually produced. As he becomes more skilled, the pause is shortened and, as with Van Riper's method, the end result is a slightly slower version of normal speech. Mainly for this reason, modification seems to be one of the most acceptable methods of control to the speakers themselves. However, it demands the utmost patience and concentration and is more appropriately applied to more severe blocks, prolongations and repetitions. Milder disruptions are quickly over and modification probably takes too long to feel effective.

Not all therapists, of course, believe in attempting to control the overt symptoms so directly. Most advocate relaxing the tension and the struggle against impending disfluency. Sheehan (1970), however, even seems to see a danger in controlling stuttering, as if it were yet another form of avoidance, allied to the 'false' fluency of trying to hide the stutter. His basic therapy procedures include exploring every aspect of the disorder and reducing the struggle, but the emphasis is on being open about it—learning to stutter in front of others 'openly and easily', seeking out feared words and situations 'instead of just letting them happen to you'. He describes his approach as 'role therapy', since he views stuttering as 'a false-role disorder—a role-specific conflict involving approach and avoidance, involving attitudinal and motoric aspects'. To Johnson (1939) the question of how one is to change the overt behaviour is not important and he, too, places the emphasis on what lies behind this behaviour. It seemed to him that 'a behaviour, in so far as it is modifiable, can be altered either directly or indirectly through changes in the assumptions which underlie the behaviour' (171). He believes that 'you can quite literally talk a stutterer into the conviction that he is able to speak more fluently than he does . . . or we can . . . tell the stutterer to behave in some way different from his customary behaviour. So far as he succeeds in following directions of this kind and finds himself exhibiting new types of behaviour, he will in time express a corresponding change in his assumptions regarding his possibilities for action' (172).

Although Johnson's view is a shrewd one with some truth in it, it would seem to us that it *does* matter how you attempt to modify the stutterer's behaviour, overt and covert; but it is at the same time quite clear that no one method is appropriate to all stutterers. Sheehan (1970, 294) expresses this well when he speaks of 'the Smorgesbord of stuttering therapy'. In this 'a variety of techniques is made available and the client tastes, rejects or accepts, based on his indiviudal inclinations. One man's favourite dish is anathema to another.' There is obvious danger of confusion if the stutterer jumps from one method to another, never going deeply enough into one technique to allow it to become established. But in any one clinic where a number of stutterers are treated, there is a clear need to have available more than one approach. One client, especially if his problem is severe, may need a strongly supporting technique such as syllable-timed speech at least for a period, while another may be able to work directly on some form of modification immediately. A very rapid speaker may find a vast improvement merely from some means of slowing down, but maintaining this slower rate of speech outside the clinical situation will need a great deal of determination and practice.

We spoke earlier of the need for all stutterers, whatever overt symptoms they manifest, to work on the psychological aspects of the disorder. This, as we have said, may entail some form of psychotherapy. In many cases, however, a simpler exploration of attitudes towards their difficulty and communication as a whole may produce a gradual necessary change. Group work provides a very useful setting for discussion, the establishment of realistic aims and desensitization, aimed at the reduction of the negative emotional factors involved for most stutterers. The group seems to provide, on the one hand, a permissive atmosphere, in which disfluency is accepted and, on the other, the support that is needed for the difficult task of controlling that disfluency. Motivation and attention can easily flag in the stutterer who is working on his own. The group is a source of encouragement and, if it is working well, of continual challenge to set attitudes, more appropriate than that provided by a fluent therapist alone. Individual therapy, though extremely valuable and probably more beneficial for some, has its limitations in the narrowness of the one-to-one communication situation. The stutterer usually finds his greatest difficulties in the face of a larger social group and the therapy group to some extent forms a bridge to the world outside the clinic. Intensive group therapy, such as the four-week courses held at the City Literary Institute in London, has a great deal to offer. Work can be taken more deeply and problems carried through from day to day. They must, however, be followed by a considerable period of therapy to establish what has been learned and to allow for change to take place more fully over time.

A recent and extremely interesting approach to the psychological dimension of stuttering, which entails individual work and stresses this need for time in the processes of change is that described by Fransella (1972). Based on Kelly's Personal Construct Theory (1955) it is aimed at helping the stutterer to reconstrue his world in terms of his 'fluent' self, rather than seeing it narrowly through the eyes of a stutterer. Briefly, Fransella believes that the stutterer experiences his disfluency so much more vividly than his fluency that all his reactions towards communication and society are governed by the disorder. She attempts to focus attention on fluency and strengthen the construct 'me as a fluent speaker', thereby weakening the overriding implications of 'me as a stutterer'. She found that fluency increased as the fluent self became more meaningful and, over a period of work, the stutterer's approach to life became closer and closer to that of a normally fluent person. Fransella herself questions whether 'such a rigorous adherence to the psychological rather than the behavioural aspects of stuttering is most advantageous for all stutterers' (230) and, like any other approach, we feel that though it could be of great benefit to some, for others it would have little value. It would be extremely difficult for a very severe stutterer, for example, to produce enough experience of fluency to reconstrue. Here, some parallel work on the overt symptoms themselves would seem essential. Not all stutterers would be able or willing to verbalize constructs in the manner proposed, this being not simply a matter of intelligence but of interest.

Fransella's ideas as to the nature of the disorder in its developed form, however, does throw some light on part of its mystery. Clinicians have been exercised over the years about the problems of the transfer of clinically achieved fluency to external situations. They see one stutterer after another master techniques of control with comparative ease, experience a genuine decrease in anxiety and shame about their speech, and yet be quite unable to bring the new speech behaviour into practice consistently in their daily lives. One simple view would be that 'old habits die hard'. Another sometimes expressed is that the stutterer clings too lovingly to the so-called 'secondary gain' that his situation affords him. A subtler one implies that the process of change entails more than the conscientious practice of new controlled patterns of speech and a more positive attitude towards communication as a whole. It also entails adjustment to the experience and responsibilities of a fluent speaker, which are very different from those of many stutterers.

Definition

In these chapters on stuttering we have considered the nature of the disorder as it first manifests itself in early childhood, and have attempted to trace its development through to the many forms manifested by the confirmed stutterer. Although it may be defined superficially as a disorder of fluency characterized by disruptions to the normal timing of speech patterns, having said that, we have said very little. More importantly, it is a disorder which, in its later forms at least, involves the speaker in anticipation, struggle and reaction to the disruptions and may impose severe restrictions on communication as a whole. Stuttering, though in many cases immediately recognizable, is very difficult to define, since no definition can encompass all its facets or express adequately each of the many complex forms in which it is presented. It is to be hoped, however, that we have managed to convey something of this complexity and its effects on communication for the speakers and the listeners involved.

8

Cluttering and disfluency of organic origin

In our earlier chapters we referred to disorders other than stuttering manifesting disfluency features. In this chapter we shall discuss such disorders in detail. Since we have maintained throughout that the term stuttering encompasses many different forms of disfluency, it may seem unnecessary to devote a section of this book to the particular type of disfluency known as cluttering. In the American and British literature, relatively little attention has been paid to it, beyond descriptions of the typically hurried and often unintelligible speech pattern produced by this group of speakers. Some European speech pathologists, however, have discussed its origins and characteristics at great length. Writers such as Froeschels, Freund, Luchsinger and, above all, Weiss, have not only outlined the disorder in detail but, less fortunately, contrasted 'the clutterer' and 'the stutterer' in terms of personality and behaviour in a way which takes no account of the wide variety and complexity of factors involved in stuttering and reduces all clutterers to a stereotype. But, while such generalization is unacceptable, there is no doubt that cluttering is a quite distinct type of disfluency and the evidence as to its possible organic basis and its special nature should be discussed.

The etiology of cluttering

Weiss (1964, 7) maintains that although 'in typical cluttering there are no neurological symptoms', the symptoms present have 'an organic flavour'. Many writers have noted its likeness to the speech of some patients suffering from Parkinson's disease, clearly organic in nature. What some have referred to as 'organic stuttering', which results sometimes from neurological disease, Weiss prefers to call 'symptomatic cluttering'. He suggests that 'any kind of brain damage—traumatic, infectious, tumoral etc.—can upset language function and produce cluttering-like symptoms' (65). Seeman (1951) attributes the symptoms of cluttering to the anomalous activity of the extrapyramidal centres. He does not, however, produce any hard evidence for this. Luchsinger and Landholt (1951) compared the EEGs of stutterers and clutterers and found that almost 90 per cent of the clutterers showed abnormalities.

One of the most extensive studies of both stutterers and clutterers, aimed at clarifying the possible organic basis for the latter, is found in Langová and Morávek (1964). They compared the two groups for EEG results, reactions to delayed auditory feedback and the effects of the drugs chlorpromazine (CLP) and dexfenmetrazine. Like Luchsinger and Landholt, they found that a high number of clutterers showed EEG abnormalities (but 50 per cent as against the earlier investigators' 90 per cent) as against 15–16 per cent of the stutterers. Of the 28 clutterers subjected to DAF, 25 showed 'expressive speech aggravation' (291). Speech was slowed down and there were many repetitions and errors. Voice became monotonous, prosody disturbed and the clutterers described 'very unpleasant feelings when speaking'. Fifty-four of the 59 stutterers examined, on the other hand, became fluent under these conditions. Eleven of the 13 clutterers taking CLP improved in speech, while 2 showed no difference. None of the 12 stutterers taking the drug improved; in fact, 8 became more disfluent. With the administration of dexfenmetrazine, the opposite results were obtained; all 8 clutterers in this experiment became worse, while 15 of the 17 stutterers improved their speech and 2 showed no effect.

Langová and Morávek consider these results to indicate a definite connection between cluttering and 'an organic or functional anomaly' (294). They base this conclusion on the abnormality of the EEGs and the positive effect on the clutterers' speech of a drug which tranquillized them, as against the negative effect of a stimulant. The fact that in this particular experiment only 50 per cent of the clutterers showed abnormal EEGs somewhat weakens their argument as to the importance of this finding, as compared with that of Luchsinger and Landholt. And while 8 of their 12 stutterers became more disfluent under CLP, Beech and Fransella (1968), from their study of the effects of drug therapy, describe chlorpromazine as the most promising of the tranquillizing drugs in reducing the frequency of stuttering. Langová and Morávek could not explain why clutterers should have reacted to DAF in a way similar to normal speakers. Because of the high number of stutterers who improved under this condition, they suggest that their difficulty is due to a clash between acoustic and proprioceptive feedback information which is one possibility put forward by Van Riper (1971) (see chapter 6). On the whole, the study would seem to do more to perpetuate the contrasting of 'the clutterer' with 'the stutterer' than to offer any clear organic evidence for cluttering.

Arnold (1960), Weiss (1964) and Luchsinger (1970), all emphasize the hereditary factor in the etiology of cluttering, which they maintain is even stronger than with other types of disfluency. Arnold declares that 'hereditary influences are prominent in most cases of cluttering speech' and that all previous authors and recent investigators 'agree on the genetic basis of this constitutional disability' (27). Weiss claims to have found not only familial cluttering but evidence of other language and behavioural disorders in the relatives of his cluttering patients, which he believes stem from a common denominator, namely a 'central language imbalance'. This he postulates as the basis not only of cluttered speech but of delayed language, dyslalias, reading and writing difficulties, disorders of rhythm and musicality and a general disorderliness and restlessness. He admits that there are no pathological anatomic findings in central language imbalance, and is at pains to separate those suffering from this underlying 'inborn weakness' from others with definable neurological disease. The clutterer he sees as 'under-endowed', while the organic case is 'incapacitated' (8).

Throughout his book, Weiss bases his theories on 'clinical observation' and 'long therapeutic experience'. He regrets that systematic research is meagre and complains of the lack of attention to cluttering, particularly in the American literature. He gives as one reason for this neglect the fact that the majority of clutterers do not seek professional help; and he cannot estimate the extent of cluttering in the general population. We also can only discuss his and his colleagues' theories in the light of clinical observation, and while we are in agreement as to the existence of this very distinct group of speakers, with clearly definable speech symptoms, our therapeutic experience does not allow us to accept either the underlying implications of a central language imbalance or the other attributes of the so-called cluttering personality. We should admit, however, that we have worked with a far greater number of clients who are what Freund (1952) referred to as stutter-clutterers, that is, showing stuttering symptoms on a cluttering basis, and with only comparatively few 'pure clutterers'. Whether these latter are indeed rare or whether they do not present for treatment, we shall probably never know.

Van Riper (1954, 25) describes cluttering as 'characterized by slurred and omitted syllables, by improper phrasing and pauses, due to excessive speed'. Luchsinger (1970, 244) sees the repetition of syllables and words as the most important feature, and remarks on 'an imperfection in finding words' amongst these speakers and 'a striking monotony of speech melody'. Weiss (1964, ch. 2) outlines the speech symptoms in greater detail. Excessive speed (tachylalia) has always been considered the most significant feature of cluttering, but he maintains with Froeschels (1946) that they only speak 'relatively too quickly' for their ability to find words and formulate sentences. 'Drawling and interjections' he sees as resulting from this difficulty. The unintelligibility of the speech of many clutterers is caused by:

(a)   omission of sounds, syllables and whole words
(b)   displacement of sounds
(c)   inversion of the order of sounds
(d)   anticipation of sounds
(e)   postposition of sounds
(f)   repetition of initial sounds
(g)   telescoping of several syllables of a word

Many of these features, including the anticipation of sounds, the postposition of sounds and the telescoping of several syllables of a word, seem to be an exaggeration of the coarticulation and elision of normal speech discussed in chapter 3. All these articulatory deviations improve when speed is reduced and, indeed, may disappear altogether. Weiss also notes the clutterer's 'jerky respiration and short respiratory span' and the monotony of the speech-melody pattern (presumably referring to intonation and pitch range). Wohl (1970) describes the prominent feature of cluttering as festinating (i.e. becoming faster and faster as speech proceeds), which leads to 'elision', articulation disorders of an erratic and unstructured type, omission and consequent spelling and writing errors. Strikingly, she says of this form of disfluency, 'It is our belief that language imbalance, contrary to traditional opinion, is resultant, not causative.'

It will be seen, then, that there is broad agreement as to the speech symptoms of cluttering, if not as to its cause. Where we do question the validity of Weiss's observations, however, is in his listing of other attributes characteristic of those who produce such a speech pattern. His first heading in this section (32) is 'lack of rhythm and musical ability', and yet he admits to knowing clutterers who, despite dysrhythmic speech, have an excellent sense of rhythm in other respects. Also, although 'poor pitch and poor sense of melody are often found with cluttering . . . some clutterers have a good sense of the musical elements' (32). This sounds like a description of the general population as a whole.

'Poor concentration and short attention span' are claimed as 'the basic symptomatic elements of cluttering' (33), but the evidence he cites for this is slight. We have known some with cluttered speech who show these difficulties, but just as many others who do not. Perhaps, as with stuttering, we should think in terms of subgroups of clutterers, showing different clusters of factors involved in their symptomatology. Liebmann (1900, 1930) proposed two groups, one being motor in form and having lack of attention to kinesthetic and somato-motor performance as its basis, while the second was said to be receptive in nature, with disorders of auditory attention predominating. Froeschels (1946) was one of the earliest to relate cluttering to a disturbance of thinking. He described the sequence of preparatory steps before a phrase or sentence is uttered: 'There is a psychic urge or attitude toward expressing a thought. This is followed by a planning of the sequence and choice of words to be expressed. Finally, the phrase or sentence is spoken' (31). (In chapter 2 we have presented a more detailed discussion of the neurological factors involved in the production of a speech utterance.) He believed that verbal expression is dependent upon these phases and that 'When an incongruity occurs between the urge to utter an idea on the one hand and the thought accomplishment and the speech accomplishment on the other, the result may be cluttering' (31). Weiss declares that the clutterer's thought is poorly integrated and incomplete. We, like Wohl, however, have found more often that it is the speed of speech which disturbs the flow of thought and, when speed is reduced, the thoughts of most seem to be as well ordered as those of normally fluent speakers. This suggests some impairment of the normal neural pacemaker discussed in chapter 2 (p. 14).

Reading disability is next said by Weiss to be characteristic of clutterers and, while it is true that in reading aloud at their habitual rate many of these speakers make a number of errors, the improvement when slowing down is often marked and reveals no basic difficulty in either pronunciation or interpretation. Similarly, the writing disorder noted by some authorities would seem to stem rather from haste than the 'reduced motor skill' attributed to clutterers by Weiss (42). Only one cluttering child in our experience showed what might be considered truly dysgraphic errors. Many others with festinant speech, however, have written carelessly and somewhat illegibly, as we all do at times. Weiss says that the clutterer's grammar is poor in speech and writing but, again, grammatical as well as articulatory errors are usually eliminated when the clutterer reduces the speed of utterance and writing.

With Weiss's point about the clutterer's lack of awareness of his symptoms we are largely in agreement. While some of these speakers are able to describe quite clearly what happens when their speech deteriorates, many just do not realize the speed at which they are speaking and are genuinely puzzled by their listeners' failure to understand them. Speed, like vocal intensity, is very difficult to judge subjectively. Many clutterers (especially those who have no stuttering component in their disorder) experience none of the anticipation of difficulty which is common to most stutterers. They may feel a little apprehensive about certain situations where they have often performed inadequately, but they do not have specific word or sound fears. If there really were disordered thought behind their disordered speech, awareness of difficulty would surely be more common.

We have also found, with Weiss and others, that many with cluttered speech are somewhat hyperactive in other ways and rather restless. Their movements are often (though not invariably) quick and they tend to react immediately to stimuli of any kind. Many fast speakers with normal fluency behave in a similar way and most of us do at some time when excited or in a hurry. It is not surprising that clutterers were found to react positively to CLP, which would calm any hyperactivity. What *is* puzzling is that the stutterers in Langová and Morávek's experiments did not also benefit. They have been shown to do so in other trials with this and other tranquillizing agents. That they did react positively to the stimulating dexfenmetrazine, which would be expected to increase tension, is even more astonishing.

The personality of the clutterer

If it were not for the fact that Weiss and his colleagues contrast the personality of the stutterer with the clutterer in a way which we know to be completely unsubstantiated, we might have more faith in the picture of the clutterer's personality presented by them, since they have apparently had a much greater experience than we of pure clutterers. But we cannot believe that this group of speakers is any more likely to fall into so generalized a pattern than the majority of stutterers. Freund (1952), in the admitted absence of research into the personality of clutterers, sets out 'a preliminary schematic comparison between certain known personality characteristics of "pure" (typical) stutterers and clutterers and the mixed stutter-clutterers':

Pure stutterers	Pure clutterers	Stutter-clutterers
Timid	Aggressive	'Mixed' personalities
Restricted	Expansive	containing features of both
Restrained	Extroverted	preceding categories
Introspective	Impulsive	
Compulsive	Uncontrolled	
Overinhibited	Hasty	
Hesitant	Overproductive	
Retarded		

Weiss (1964) goes into even more detail about personality attributes of the clutterer. They show, he says, 'impatience, superficiality, casual acceptance of life, lack of consideration of the consequences of a given act or for other people and a short temper which is easily placated'. Moreover, they are 'poor listeners' and 'under-achievers'.

In his discussion of differential diagnosis from stuttering (he prefers the term 'stammering') Weiss adds some further generalizations in his list of 'typical differences' between the two. Some describe speech behaviour, others, again, touch on personality.

	Cluttering	*Stammering*
Awareness of disorder	Absent	Present
Speaking under stress	Better	Worse
Speaking in relaxed situation	Worse	Better
Calling attention to speech	Better	Worse
Speaking after interruption	Better	Worse
Short answers	Better	Worse
Foreign language	Better	Worse
Reading a well-known text	Worse	Better
Reading an unknown text	Better	Worse
Handwriting	Hasty, repetitious, uninhibited	Contracted, forced, inhibited
Attitude towards own speech	Careless	Fearful
Psychological attitude	Outgoing	Rather withdrawn
Aptitude (academic)	Under-achiever	Good to superior
EEG	Often diffuse dysrhythmia	Usually normal
Goal of therapy	Directing attention to speech details	Directing attention from speech details

Amongst the points under 'stammering' we would dispute that 'calling attention to speech' makes disfluency worse, or that 'short answers' are always worse than longer utterances. Not all stutterers are worse when speaking foreign languages—often the contrary. Nor is the handwriting of all stutterers 'contracted, forced, inhibited'. Their academic aptitude may be poor as well as 'good to superior'· And we would by no means agree that the goal of therapy with stuttering should be 'diverting attention from speech details'. While we admit to less experience with pure clutterers, we are not much happier with the list under 'cluttering'. Awareness of the disorder may be absent in some, but by no means all. They are not, on the whole, better while speaking under stress. We have not found them better at reading an unknown text than a well-known text. Only one or two of those with whom we have worked have had a careless attitude towards their own speech and, as far as we can judge, none have been 'under-achievers'. We would agree, however, that 'directing attention to speech details' is one very important goal of therapy.

The relationship between cluttering and stuttering

Freund (1952) describes the early disfluencies of small children as 'physiologic' stuttering or cluttering. He relates the 'incongruence between liveliness of speech-drive and the limited infantile ability of word-finding and inner formulation' (148) in children to the disfluency of older clutterers. The typical repetitive features of early nonfluency can certainly be related, but we did not find in our study in chapter 5 either the excessive speed or the resultant articulatory deviations leading to unintelligibility in this early stage of speech development. To Froeschels and also Weiss, cluttering is not only a speech disturbance in its own right, but also the primary basis of much stuttering. Discussions by these authors on the relationship between stuttering and cluttering presupposes the three groups referred to by Freund (1952): 'pure' stutterers, 'pure' clutterers and stutter-clutterers. The latter are said to develop from cluttering, to show mixed characteristics of the other two groups and to require therapeutic approaches which combine attention to both components.

Langová and Morávek (1964) included a group of stuttering clutterers in their experiments described earlier. The results, as we might expect, present a mixed picture. Thirty-nine per cent of them showed abnormal EEGs, 23 per cent improved under DAF, 55 per cent became more disfluent and 22 per cent showed no influence. Their reaction to CLP was similar to that of the pure clutterers: 8 of the 11 improved, 1 became worse and 2 did not change. Under dexfenmetrazine, 7 became more disfluent and 4 remained unaffected. Although we find Freund's reference to his stutter-clutterers having 'mixed' personalities containing features of the other two groups rather difficult to understand, and feel (as with the others) that character and behaviour cannot be tabulated, we do find this grouping to be quite valid. Wohl (1970) estimates that the disfluent speakers she describes as 'festinating' represent 25 per cent of those requiring treatment, and we would agree that of those attending the Speech Therapy Unit of the City Literary Institute in London, about a quarter have this underlying difficulty, i.e. are probably stuttering clutterers.

Van Riper's track II presents a comprehensive outline of the nature and development of this type of stuttering (see chapter 6, p. 87). He notes that fluency disruptions develop early in the speech of these children and that the onset of stuttering comes with the onset of connected speech. They have more difficulty than his track I speakers at this stage but show, on the whole, less frustration. Van Riper feels that these children could be viewed as clutterers early on, but later 'they certainly show all the characteristics of true stuttering'. Their disfluency may well have emerged from pure cluttering, but they 'end up as stutterers. They do not become fluent when they try to talk slowly and carefully. They eventually become aware of their disordered speech . . . and they develop some rare but real situation and phonemic fears. They talk in torrents. They use avoidance tricks and consider themselves stutterers' (Van Riper 1971, 111).

Effects of cluttering on communication for speaker and listener

If, as Weiss maintains, many pure clutterers do not feel the need for treatment of their speech disorder, clearly the effects on communication for them are minimal. Some of those with whom we have worked, however, *are* concerned, and one or two have shown real anxiety about their failure to speak effectively, especially in relation to the needs of their work situation. Although one recently admitted that he had felt it was 'the listeners' problem' in the past when there was some misunderstanding, he had come for treatment because of what he described as an 'uneasiness' about his speech. He could not pinpoint what was wrong, but realized that, on many occasions, he had completely failed to convey either information or his feelings about something with the clarity that he desired. He is a 'pure' clutterer, with all the classical speech symptoms but, while he has not developed the avoidances and fear of many adult stutterers, he is by no means 'careless' in his attitude towards his speech.

Others have come for treatment with little anxiety, but some frustration at not being understood. Often, the initial suggestion has come from someone else but, on the whole, once the nature of the problem has been clarified, the clutterer has realized his listener's difficulty and the need for some effort on his part. Several of our clutterers who have worked with us in recent years have come from India or Pakistan and, while we have done no research into this area, there would seem to be a cultural factor here, related perhaps to the rhythmic patterns of their first language. It might be worth while to investigate the relationship between the type of disfluencies produced by speakers of a number of different languages and aspects of those languages, such as rhythm and complexity of articulatory patterns.

Whatever the degree of concern amongst the clutterers themselves, however, there is no doubt that communication can be seriously affected for their listeners. Though there are typically no associated movements or facial contortions for them to adjust to, the effect of the speed and, more particularly, the unintelligibility of this speech pattern at its most severe, can cause tension in the listener, frustration and even confusion. A great deal of concentration is often demanded, simply to follow what a clutterer is saying, and in shorter utterances many repetitions may be needed before a request, for example, can be complied with. One of our clients used to have the greatest difficulty ordering drinks in the local pub—not because he was apprehensive, but because he ran his request for 'a pint of special' into what sounded like a single word, completely unintelligible to those serving. Another took some time to realize that his full name, containing one word of two and one of three syllables, emerged as a single word of two syllables, unrecognizable to an English speaker. True, the listeners are usually spared the anxiety transmitted by many stutterers, but they often produce their own in their effort to grasp the clutterer's meaning.

The treatment of cluttering

Froeschels (1946) had some very clear ideas as to the appropriate treatment for cluttering:

> The primary aim is towards the right order in line between the thought phase and speech phase. Since the speech phase is more accessible to the speech therapist than would be the thought phase, those devices are used which help the patient to control the accuracy, and therefore the tempo, of his articulation.

Froeschels used as one of these devices a pictorial phonetic script, which consisted of 'a series of alphabetical drawings of the most characteristic portions of the speech mechanism (e.g. lips, teeth, tongue, nose) in their positions at the time of enunciating particular sounds. The patient is asked to transcribe reading passages into this phonetic alphabet at frequent intervals daily.' He also found that clutterers benefited from lipreading and indicating the place of articulation in reading and conversation. He claimed that 'every case treated in this way so far could be cured within three to six months'.

Weiss used a number of methods with clutterers: syllabization (similar to the syllable-timed speech described in chapter 7), rhythmical tapping, shadowing exercises and other activities based on reading, including reading letter by letter. Phonetic transcription he has found useful and, more surprisingly, reading backwards. We can see that this would undoubtedly have the effect of slowing the reader down, but not the connection between this and the control of normal speech. Exaggerated accentuation of stressed syllables is also practised and work done on vocabulary and formulation. The repetition of stories, which Weiss says they find very difficult, is developed throughout treatment. To help them extend their poor attention span and concentration they are asked to count backwards.

We have found syllable-timed speech very useful in the early stages of treatment with cluttering, since it discourages the elision and extensive coarticulation of syllables and words, and inevitably slows the rate of speech. Often, however, simply slowing down has a marked effect, and it is maintaining this slower speed outside the clinic which proves the problem. Certainly, the clutterer's main task is to develop a fuller awareness of his speech pattern and an effective means of monitoring his speech consciously using the neurosensory feedback channels mentioned in chapter 2. Though this may easily be achieved in the context of therapy sessions, it takes a great deal of self-discipline to transfer these abilities to everyday life. Weiss believes that the prognosis is poor for many clutterers. We have found variable results and, as with the treatment of all kinds of disfluency, the key factor seems to lie in the determination and sheer hard work of the particular clutterer.

Disfluency in Parkinson's disease

We mentioned earlier that reference is often made to the similarity between cluttering and the speech of some patients suffering from Parkinson's disease.

Indeed, it is this likeness, rather than the evidence so far, which causes many workers to feel that cluttering may have an organic basis. Greene (1964, 227) describes the speech of post-encephalitic Parkinsonism as 'slurred, monotonous and quavery, with a tendency to accelerate and trail away'. Unlike clutterers, however, these patients show 'lack of speech propulsion or initiative', the voice is 'weak and tremulous and fades away or deteriorates into a palilalic murmur'. Clutterers are generally felt to have a characteristic 'liveliness of speech drive' (Freund 1952) and although often similarly lacking in intonation, the voice itself is not typically weak or quavering. The palilalia referred to by Greene describes a series of rapid repetitions, which may be seen as a cluttering feature.

Parkinsonism results from striatal lesions, specifically lesions of the globus pallidus and substantia nigra which are important in control of movement, and disfluency is only one of the difficulties experienced by these patients. It is the rigidity of the muscles of the larynx which makes the voice weak and involvement of the articulatory muscles results in dysarthria. There may, in addition, be excessive salivation, difficulty in swallowing, and tremor of the mouth and tongue, none of which has been found amongst clutterers. Brain (1960) notes the tendency in some of these patients for writing to become smaller (micrographia), but there is no similarity between this factor and the careless scrawl of some clutterers.

There is a similar difficulty in treatment, however, of awareness of speech deterioration. Although with Parkinsonism speech therapy is aimed at maintaining communication at as high a level as possible for as long as possible, as against the attempt to control the symptoms of cluttering, there is the same primary need in both approaches to develop a greater sensitivity in the speaker to acceleration and reduction of precision in articulation. Many patients find it extremely difficult to monitor their speech behaviour, and while they too can produce far greater clarity in 'speech exercises', it is easily lost in ordinary conversation. For some, especially in the later stages of the disease, the effort required for control is simply too great, and the dysphonic component, which clutterers do not share, adds to the problem for the listener. Greene regards speech therapy for these patients as having a largely palliative and psychological value. She suggests that in the early stages 'relaxation and reassurance and encouragement to speak and not relinquish the attempt may inspire a patient to make the best use of residual function'. Perhaps the greatest distinction between Parkinsonian disfluency and cluttering lies in the progressive nature of the former, while, with the latter, speech will always improve if appropriate measures are taken.

Disfluency caused by dysarthria

We referred to the articulatory difficulty in Parkinson's disease, already discussed in chapter 3, as one form of dysarthria. This term is defined by Greene (1964, 223) as 'defective articulation due to lesions in the nervous system which cause motor disorders of the muscles of articulation'. It may take one of several forms, depending on the site of the lesion, but in all cases fluency will be affected. Articulation will be imprecise or even rendered unintelligible, some sounds being distorted or omitted altogether. Intonation is often reduced by accompanying weakness of the laryngeal or respiratory muscles or prosody disturbed by the reduced range of these muscles. In spastic dysarthria, caused by damage to the upper motor neurone of the nerves involved in speech, the tension within the muscles may be too strong at the beginning of a phrase and then fade away. Low vital capacity, causing shallowness of respiration and lack of coordination between phonation and respiration may cause further disruption. (See chapter 3 for discussion of the relationship of these three physiological systems involved in speech production.) Other striatal lesions besides those causing Parkinson's disease will also produce a characteristic type of dysarthria. In athetosis, articulation and voice may be disrupted by involuntary movements of the respiratory muscles, larynx and tongue. Appropriate pitch changes and stress may be lost altogether. In cases of chorea, rapid, jerky involuntary movements of the muscles of the face, tongue palate and larynx make the normal flow of speech impossible. Lesions of the brain-stem produce a flaccid paralysis and wasting in the muscles used in swallowing, articulation and phonation. Greene describes the resultant speech pattern as 'slow and laboured, the voice hollow and uninflected . . . the muscles tire quickly, so that isolated words may be just recognizable, but a phrase deteriorates into laboured and undifferentiated phonation' (230). With damage to the cerebellum, muscle tone is reduced and ataxia, a disorder of coordination and balance, results. The fine coordination needed for clear articulation becomes impossible and speech is slurred, slow and hesitant. Rhythm and phonation, according to Peacher (1950), are often more impaired than articulation itself. Disseminated sclerosis often entails this type of disfluency.

Clearly the dysarthrias are different in origin and nature from the disfluencies we have discussed at greater length. They are primarily defects of phonetic transition, where neurological impairment prevents the execution of precise articulatory target movements, with the additional factors of loss of intonation and stress further affecting communication. Children suffering from cerebral palsy frequently have dysarthria among their other motor disorders and some of them are never able to communicate effectively. When this occurs in adults, as one result of neurological disease, a 'stroke' or an accident, they may become very distressed by their inability to speak with their accustomed ease and clarity. For the listener, severely dysarthric speech may prove a complete barrier to understanding and often the disordered speech is taken to represent loss of intellect. So radical a change in speech behaviour may give the impression of a changed personality, though this is seldom the case. Treatment must be aimed not only at encouraging the patient to achieve and maintain the highest possible level of articulation, but, just as important, at helping those round him to adjust to changes in many aspects of behaviour.

Treatment of dysarthria

Treatment of dysarthric disfluency will to some extent vary according to the type and origin of the disorder. But one or two generalizations can be made in principle.

A careful assessment must first be made of the involvement of the muscles of the speech mechanism in terms of the paralysis, weakness, incoordination or involuntary movement caused by the brain lesion. The effects on respiration, phonation and articulation must be measured, noting specific losses in breath control and phrasing, pitch control, volume, intonation, speech rhythm and speed control, as well as details of the resultant omissions, substitutions, elisions and imprecisions of phonetic segments. Since all these elements vary according to context, the assessment must include all levels, from the production of single sounds to conversational speech, and the point of breakdown be noted for each feature.

Therapy may range from the restoration of muscular activity through exercise, stimulation with an electric brush and stroking with ice (see Draper 1968) to the maintenance of appropriate intonation and speed in spontaneous conversation through the development of self-monitoring and conservation of energy. In very severe cases, alternative means of communication through writing or signing may be necessary. In mild cases, conscious attention to precise articulation may be the main aim. For many speakers, work is built up from the achievement of appropriate placement of single sounds to their use in ever-increasing units, together with the restoration of stress and rhythm and the development of phrasing according to breath capacity and control. For them, too, self-monitoring is all-important. Whatever the severity, we are aiming at the most effective communication possible to each person and our concern must be with the satisfaction of both speaker and listener.

Articulatory dyspraxia

Defined at its simplest as an inability to perform purposeful movements in the absence of paralysis, dyspraxia has for some time been the subject of controversy in speech pathology. People suffering from this disability can be seen to struggle to produce speech in a way which sometimes looks and sounds like stuttering. But there the similarity ends. The dyspraxic speaker may, like the stutterer, know exactly what he wants to say and be unable to speak with ease, but the cause of the difficulty lies in his failure to make the appropriate contacts and movements required to produce the sounds he wants to form particular words. Although the problem may increase under stress, there is nothing like the variability of stuttering and the patient is never free from dyspraxia. Darley, Aronson and Brown (1969a) speak of 'a faulty programming of movements and sequences of movements for speech'. While they see it as something more complex than Wepman's 'disturbance on the output side below the level of meaning', they clearly approach it as a difficulty on the motor side of speech and language. Other writers, however, have been dissatisfied with such a concept. They note that dyspraxia very rarely occurs without other aphasic impairment—that is other effects which are linguistic, not purely motor in nature. Just as some aphasic people substitute one word for another, so the dyspraxic substitutes one sound for another. The sequencing of speech sounds is disrupted in dyspraxia, just as the sequencing of words and morphemes may be disrupted in aphasia. The basic difficulty of selection common to most dysphasic speakers is reflected in dyspraxia in a difficulty in selecting phonemes.

Martin (1974) rejects the term dyspraxia of speech because of the implications of a purely mechanical failure, as in dypraxia of limbs, and prefers the phrase 'aphasic phonological impairment'. The word 'phonological' pinpoints the aspect of speech under consideration, while 'aphasic' differentiates it from other articulatory disorders—in particular dysarthria. Whether we regard dyspraxia as a purely motor or a more complex linguistic disability, however, fluency may be affected by even a mild degree and completely destroyed by severe dyspraxia (or apraxia). The transitions between sound segments and syllables are slow and laboured, and the phonological system may be reduced to a few sounds only. Normal intonation patterns may be altered and pitch range reduced or retained to some extent, depending on severity. And in many cases the flow of speech is further hindered by other aphasic problems, such as word-finding difficulty or disturbed formulation. The speaker is often only too aware of his errors and may make many attempts at self-correction. Frustration can be extreme and, unlike most stutterers, the patient suffering from acquired dyspraxia (due, for instance, to a 'stroke') has not had a lifetime to adjust to disfluency.

The dyspraxic child is in a rather different situation. From the beginnings of speech some children have this problem and they learn to produce their own patterns of sound, which do not match those of the speakers round them, but which they accept as appropriate. They have to learn to discriminate between their sounds and those made by other speakers and gradually to approximate their system to that of their fellows. The adult dyspraxic, however, remembers how the sounds should be and must learn again how to make them accurately. The prognosis for dyspraxia depends largely on severity and on how much spontaneous recovery takes place, allowing a freer flow of speech. Where the condition remains severe for a considerable time after the causal illness, it may be very hard labour indeed to produce old sounds anew and the speaker may never regain fluency.

Treatment of dyspraxia

It will be clear that approaches to the restoration of fluency for the dyspraxic speaker will differ greatly from those briefly outlined for dysarthria. Here there is no weakness to be strengthened. At the simplest level, the power of movement is there but misdirected, and our task is to help the speaker to re-establish appropriate articulatory patterns for producing and sequencing speech sounds. Careful assessment will again show us the extent to which speech is affected, from the single-sound level to connected, conversational speech. One essential aspect of assessment which has been very largely neglected, at least in the textbooks, is an evaluation of the patient's response to different types of cueing. This, in itself, holds clear indications for treatment. In one case, for instance, a speaker may be unable to utter a single word spontaneously, but when given the initial sound of the first word required, goes on to produce a whole phrase. Another, with rather more, though laboured, spontaneous speech at his command, may have to watch and imitate each segment of a new phrase, suggesting that he is organizing each set of movements, step by step as he speaks. The two are clearly quite distinct types of dyspraxia. The first is a total loss of what might be called articulatory memory, which can be stimulated by a single cue. The second suggests a very definite interference with attempts to position the articulators, which can only be overcome by a conscious effort made with the help of a strong stimulus to imitate.

These are just two examples of differences in the type of problem the speaker is experiencing. It is not surprising, therefore, that therapeutic approaches vary widely amongst the authorities. And it is certain that no one method will suit every case of dyspraxia. It may be necessary for therapy to begin at the most basic level of eliciting phonation. This can be done by extending natural sounds, such as laughing and coughing. Schuell, Jenkins and Jimenez-Pabon (1964) also suggest placing the hand lightly on the patient's larynx and asking him to 'push hard'—an effort which invariably produces vocal sound. This is then varied by prolongation and changes in volume and pitch. Most workers advocate next the elicitation of vowels and other 'visible' sounds, which can be imitated directly or by the use of a mirror for watching the therapist's lips, as well as monitoring the patient's own movements. Luria (1970, 388 ff) uses natural movements as a basis, such as blowing out a match on /p/, and presents his patients with articulatory diagrams, showing the position of the lips, tongue and teeth for particular phrases. Schuell, on the other hand, works from whole words by stimulating singing, serial speech and associative speech, as in phrases such as 'bread and ——', 'a cup of ——', which are often available to these patients.

It will be noticed that the emphasis is not on phonetic placement but on automatic speech and visual cues, with auditory monitoring. Patients seldom respond to direct instructions to 'place the tongue-tip on the upper teeth ridge', for example, since that is exactly what they are trying and failing to do. Rosenbek et al. (1973) outline a careful programme for treatment of apraxia in adults in a series of small steps, which they describe as a 'task continuum'. Briefly, this involves the patient's watching and listening to produce direct imitation, then delayed production, with the written word and the patient's own writing to reinforce the unit of speech attempted and, lastly, the production of that unit in response to a question. Although their trial of this particular continuum was limited, some such step-by-step approach is undoubtedly necessary in many cases, but tailormade to suit a particular speaker. Once again, appropriate treatment can only be governed by the most careful analysis of specific speech deviations produced by each dyspraxic person. Not only is there undoubtedly more than one type of dyspraxia, but dyspraxic speakers within the broad groups vary from one another in the difficulty they experience, and this individuality should be kept in mind throughout any course of treatment.

Loss of fluency in dysphasia

We saw in our earlier chapters that fluency may be disturbed for the normal speaker at every level of thought and language. Confusion of ideas will frequently lead to speech characterized by hesitations, increased occurrence of pauses both filled and unfilled, and other disfluency features such as repetitions and revisions. Difficulty in formulation may present a similar picture. Momentary loss of a word leads to undue pausing, sometimes repetition. Uncertainty over pronunciation can produce repetition of syllables or sounds, as well as whole words. In many cases of dysphasia, all these essentially normal difficulties may be exaggerated, with a serious effect on fluency of speech as well as on other aspects of expression.

The most fluent dysphasic speaker is often the most handicapped. With loss of auditory verbal perception, the person affected may produce an uninterrupted flow of jargon where intonation is intact. Although this may be different in nature from the jargon of early childhood, having usually a wider range of sound and syllable combinations, it is interesting to remember that in childhood, too, jargon is never disfluent. The dyspraxic people discussed above, who have other aphasic symptoms, may (though never fluent when attempting true speech) have uninterrupted phrases of stereotyped greeting or recurrent utterance of a possibly meaningful but inappropriate phrase. Some patients quite seriously affected in both comprehension and word-finding may be relatively fluent in circumlocution, though on the whole this type of speech is slow and hesitant.

In most other cases, however, disruption of language at various levels always causes disruption of the flow of speech. The person with formulation difficulty moves slowly from word to word and phrase to phrase as he tries to express his thoughts with an inadequate grasp of syntactic structure (see chapter 3 on transition smoothness). Word-finding difficulty is perhaps the most obvious cause of disfluency amongst dysphasic speakers. At best, speech is slow, repetitive and hesitant; at worst, full of long pauses and frustrating false trials. We have discussed the phonological problems of dyspraxic people, but other difficulties related to the paraphasias can also break up the flow of speech. Verbal paraphasia is usually defined as the substitution of words sought by associated but inappropriate ones. Literal paraphasia is usually defined as the substitution of inappropriate sounds. The more aware the speaker is of his errors, the more halting his speech will be.

The most disfluent group of all is that suffering from what Luria (1970) describes as 'frontal' or 'dynamic' aphasia, where all initiative to speak is lost and the patient often cannot utter without some form of cueing. Although this difficulty is by no means common to all dysphasics, all are in some way handicapped in fluency. As they improve with treatment aimed at restoring vocabulary and the proper sequencing of words and articulatory patterns, speech in many remains slower and more hesitant than normal. They usually need more time to take in a question or statement from someone else and take longer to formulate and express their reply. In some of these people the main difficulty is in ordering their thoughts smoothly, in others formulating expression, in still others the more superficial but equally hampering pronunciation of the words needed for that expression. It is important for those who have to do with these patients to realize that time is needed sometimes for comprehension, almost always for expression. All too often a relative or friend will rush in to help, and eventually the dysphasic person may give up the struggle and remain silent.

Clearly, every kind of impairment in dysphasia affects communication for both speaker and listener. The shock to the speaker at finding himself unable to understand or express himself can only be guessed at by those who have not experienced this situation. The frustration of someone who has hitherto spoken with ease at finding himself stumbling and groping for words must be far greater than for even the severest stutterer, who has lived with his problem for some time and has at least no language disability. The relatives and friends of dysphasic people are often distressed by the change in the speaker and need time to adjust to his difficulties. As with the dysarthric, they often mistake the language loss for loss of intellect, and careful explanation as well as full information is as important for them as for the patient. When this is handled well, however, many families manage to adjust to what may be severely reduced communication. Writing, though often affected, may be used to supplement speech, and some are ingenious in developing gesture and other signs to make themselves understood. Loss of fluency in these cases is a minor problem compared with the loss of some far more important aspects of speech and language.

Treatment of dysphasia

Dysphasia will be discussed in detail in a later volume in this series, and therefore we will outline only very briefly some of the approaches to its assessment and treatment. The assessment of the multiple problems involved is a vast and complex subject in itself. No therapist seems entirely satisfied with the standardized assessments available. That of Schuell and her colleagues (1964) is perhaps the most widely used. It investigates auditory comprehension, reading, aspects of speech and language production, writing and numerical ability. It is a thorough and comprehensive set of tests, but has been criticized for the all-or-nothing scoring, which is insensitive to degrees of improvement on retesting. Others such as Eisenson's (1958) is considered not to be comprehensive enough and to give only a broad picture of aphasic impairment. What is required is a full account of the deficits and assets in the language of each patient, not just in response to test material, but in spontaneous conversation, in the context of their daily lives. Scoring needs to be subtle enough to show changes towards or away from the appropriate response, rather than simply be restricted to 'right' or 'wrong' in every aspect of language and language-linked activities.

It is on such a profile of assets and deficits, together with medical, personal and social information, that the treatment of aphasia should be based. It is usually advocated that therapists begin at the point at which the patient *can* succeed but is beginning to experience difficulty. Attempts are made to rebuild vocabulary and syntactic structure in carefully planned steps, one leading to the potential achievement of the next. For example, if a patient has lost his ability to write and can barely copy at the time of assessment, he needs to work through the stages from accurate copying, then writing the copied material from memory, to material which requires part copying, part filling-in, to very simple dictation and only later to spontaneous writing. If the person's speech is 'telegrammatic', he cannot immediately be stimulated to produce complete phrases, but must be encouraged gradually to expand his utterances to include the missing syntactic segments as they become more available to him though retraining.

Such careful, systematic work is clearly necessary for many patients, but it is not the only method that can stimulate a freer flow of language. Wepman (1972) suggests a less direct, 'context-centred' rather than 'language-centred' approach. Here the onus is on the stimulating quality of the material, and the demands made on the patient are less for accuracy than for spontaneity. By his involvement with the subject, the speaker may produce far more speech than when he is limited to finding a specific response. In group work with dysphasic people at the City Literary Institute, this kind of approach has been found to elicit a greater freedom of utterance than more highly structured material. This type of work, does, in fact, have its own structure and is far from being a simple attempt to stimulate 'talk', regardless of the quality of what is produced. The theme has to be chosen with care, with the particular patient's knowledge and interests in mind, and the therapist may need to monitor the conversation with great skill to elicit the speaker's optimum level of language.

Whatever the approach chosen as the most appropriate for particular speakers, work on dysphasia can be long and hard and the therapist's task must be to make that work meaningful, useful and genuinely interesting to the patient and those round him. She must involve the family and friends at all times, since it is they who live his life with him, and through their cooperation and understanding any treatment plans will flourish or fail.

The relationship between cluttering and organically-based disfluency

We found in the early part of this chapter that there was some evidence for the theory that cluttering is organic in origin. We are not satisfied that Weiss's central language imbalance exists, but we cannot ignore the work done by Luchsinger and Landholt (1951) when they investigated the EEGs of clutterers and stutterers and found that 90 per cent of the former showed abnormalities. The experiments of Langová and Morávek add little to the evidence. Their 50 per cent abnormal EEGs seems to leave the question more open, and the fact that clutterers behaved as normally fluent speakers under DAF conditions is uninformative. A striking likeness has been noted between cluttering and the speech of some patients suffering from Parkinson's disease, but we found considerable differences. Seeman's belief (1951) that cluttering is due to 'the anomalous activity of the extrapyramidal centres' is unsubstantiated and probably based on the likeness to Parkinsonian speech, which is of course due to extrapyramidal lesions.

Far closer to cluttering is that form of disfluency generally referred to as 'organic stuttering', which sometimes occurs as one of the sequels of brain damage, along with aphasic symptoms. Weiss calls it 'symptomatic cluttering', which may be a more appropriate term. This, to us, is what gives cluttering its 'organic flavour', but it has not been possible to isolate the lesion causing this disfluency in patients after a stroke or to compare any particular factor with clutterers as a whole. Freund (1952) contains many links made by earlier writers between stuttering and aphasia: Denhardt actually called it 'associated aphasia', while Joshimi Kaida (1930) apparently assumed in stutterers 'the existence of an aphasia-like disturbance of "proposition" ', or the ability to organize sentences. Writers on cluttering are for the most part rather less specific in their references, only speaking of 'disturbance of motor integration' suggestive of dyspraxia (de Hirsch 1961), 'word-finding difficulty' (Luchsinger 1970) and 'the dyslexia of the clutterer' (Weiss 1964, 39). But we have found that articulatory, dyslexic and indeed dysgraphic difficulties disappear when speech, reading and writing are taken at a slower rate. Weiss, however, goes on to suggest that what he calls the 'grammatical difficulties' of the clutterer 'stand astride the line which separates (or unites) the expressive and receptive realms of speech' and postulates that the 'poorly integrated thought processes and the gaps of inner language can be paralleled with transcortical aphasia'. Lack of musicality and rhythm, he says, 'bears a resemblance to amusia', a disability sometimes found with aphasia.

Since, however, we find ourselves unable to accept that even all 'pure clutterers' have these problems of grammar, inner language and lack of musicality, we do not feel that the relationship between cluttering and some aphasic impairment has really been established. A good deal more investigation needs to be done to clarify just what this particular type of disfluency stems from, and we would suggest that a comparison between clutterers and fluent, fast speakers might be more fruitful than comparisons between clutterers and stutterers, or between clutterers and those suffering from disfluency of organic origin.

9

Some indications for future work

It has been the purpose of this volume to relate disorders of fluency to ideas from many disciplines about fluency and normal nonfluency, and we have attempted throughout to assess the effects of disfluency on communication as a whole. It will be clear that our task is far from being complete. In this chapter we shall try to indicate the main gaps in our knowledge which must be filled before we can approach this aspect of language disability with any real understanding.

Various evaluations of fluency discussed in chapter 1 have been shown to lack precision and general agreement, and it would seem essential for some acceptable measures of normal fluency to be established before disfluency can be judged with confidence. Our model of speech production presented in chapter 2 is inevitably somewhat speculative, in view of our lack of detailed information on brain function. We await further research into this area and the development of techniques of investigation before a fuller account of the intricacies of speech in all its aspects can be given. Chapter 3 attempted to summarize ideas related to the temporal and sequential ordering of speech events at the output end of the encoding process and provided a basis for our discussion in later chapters of deviations from the normal ordering of this process. As we saw in this section, there is much to be learnt concerning nonfluency in normal speech.

When we come to the chapters on the disorders themselves, the inadequacy of our knowledge also manifests itself. The need for research into the nature of stuttering, cluttering and articulatory dyspraxia in particular is obvious. And none of us can be satisfied with the therapeutic measures at present available for any of the disorders. Opportunities and facilities for research in this country are extremely sparse, and even in the United States, research projects, though much more numerous, tend to be isolated from one another in their concern for separate attributes of the disfluencies, rather than aiming at the gradual building of an integrated picture of this aspect of communication.

But we shall first try to piece together the ideas about the significance of disfluent speech as an expression of personality attributes. Stuttering can, of course, lead to unintelligibility at its most severe; and some of the grosser physical and audible manifestations can distract from the content of what is being said to a large degree. We found (chapter 7) that, on the whole, stuttering did not affect the listener's impression of characteristics such as trustworthiness; but competence and dynamism, for example, were rated significantly low in these speakers. The commonly held view of the stutterer as a 'nervous' person must have some effect on the listeners' picture of stutterers as a whole and a good deal more research needs to be done in this area before those who work continually with stutterers can form a clear idea of the effect of their disfluent speech on others.

According to Weiss (1964), the clutterer's disfluency is rooted in the first ideation stage of speech production; and although we have questioned this theory as an explanation of all cluttering, there is some evidence that in those at least who show reading, writing and other problems, there may be a more basic communication difficulty than can be explained by failure at the myodynamic execution stage. We have spoken of the difficulty which many clutterers experience in monitoring, particularly the speed of their speech, and it would seem that many of them do lack the ability to make this largely automatic process a conscious one and scan their utterance sufficiently to prevent errors of elision, omission and distortion. Weiss maintains that these problems are unknown to the speaker and, therefore, do not affect communication for him. We would doubt this, as we have found far more awareness of speech inadequacy amongst clutterers, although they may not be able to say exactly what is going wrong. The effect on the listener, however, of cluttered speech is indisputable. The main result, of course, is unintelligibility where the cluttering is severe; and even in a milder form, the telescoping of words and phrases makes for somewhat tense and uneasy listening.

We know of no experimental work on the effects on communication of the dysarthrias. Our suggestions, therefore, are made from clinical observation and we feel this an area well worth investigation. In severe dysarthria, we have seen that speech can be rendered impossible. Ideas may be conveyed in writing or simple ones in gesture, but all the attributes of vocal expression conveyed by voice quality, articulation, intonation, stress and rhythm are lost. And even in less severe degrees, much of the effectiveness of these attributes is lessened. The individuality of the particular speaker is no longer distinct; in fact, one dysarthric person sounds very much like another. For each the effort to speak may be great, and many give up altogether and resort to silence and essential gesture. For some listeners, of course, knowledge of the speaker's thoughts and feelings enables them to retain their sense of the personality they have always known, but sometimes even close relatives have expressed their impression that the dysarthric person is changed, particularly intellectually. Where communication is severely reduced between members of a family, relationships may alter radically, and it is part of the therapist's task to prevent such change occurring.

We have discussed the frustration of the dyspraxic patient and the effect that failure to articulate the required sequences of target articulations may have on him. Not only is intelligibility reduced through imprecision or distortion of articulation, but intonation, stress and the natural rhythms of speech are severely disturbed. Dyspraxic speakers may struggle on, or they too may give up many attempts to communicate. Their listeners, in severe cases, may experience the greatest difficulty in understanding them and perhaps begin to avoid conversation with them to save embarrassment. Some of our clients complain that their relatives continually speak for them at home and visitors even talk across them, as if they were not present.

Once again, the speaker's role in the household may alter drastically and with it his sense of worth and responsibility.

We have commented only briefly on the subject of dysphasia, since a later volume in this series will be devoted to it and disfluency is only one aspect of this highly complex disorder. Suffice it to say that speech production may be impaired at every stage outlined earlier, with results varying from complete loss of meaning to a slight reduction in fluency. Since comprehension, too, may be affected, it will be seen that, for these patients and their listeners, the communication situation may be the most difficult of all. Dysphasia is too little understood by the experts, let alone the relatives and friends involved, and research needs in this area must include far more data as to the effects on speakers and listeners if we are to treat the disorder at all adequately.

From this brief recapitulation of such knowledge as we have concerning the effects of disorders of fluency on communication, it will be seen that it is far more than a simple matter of a loss of the natural 'flow' of speech from the speaker, with slightly more effort needed on the part of the listener to decode the message. In the severest cases of disfluency, ideation not only loses its effect at later stages of output, but can actually be disrupted for the speaker himself. Difficulties of smooth transition may lead to confusion at the neurolinguistic planning stage or produce in themselves speech which is disjointed or even unintelligible. For the listener there may be a fairly simple disturbance which interpretation of the message can easily adjust, or complete distraction from the message itself, with interference from judgements on the competence or affective state of the person trying to convey that message. We are not dealing, therefore, with the mechanical aspect of language alone but, in many cases, touching on the heart of communication between people. It is to be hoped that our few ideas will both underline the importance of this field of study and emphasize in some measure the need for further investigation. In the next section we shall attempt to indicate some of the aspects of the disorders which seem to us to demand far fuller research and understanding.

Research needs in stuttering

Stuttering is undoubtedly the most complex of the disfluencies and our lack of understanding of it begins with our ignorance of its origins. We have already indicated that many workers seem to agree that we are dealing with a number of related disorders, rather than a single one, but that attempts to divide types of stuttering into groups which hold some implications for appropriate treatment have so far failed. There are too many variables. Family history, mode and age of onset, environmental factors, attitudes, personality factors and overt and covert symptoms tend to place a particular stutterer first in one 'category', then in another. Nevertheless, it should be possible to make some distinctions, right at the beginning, in our approach to disfluency in relation to its onset. We have suggested, for instance (chapter 6), that in some cases the occurrence of disruption with the development of expressive language into connected speech shows a strong probability of a link with difficulties of formulation. Here, perhaps, instead of concerning ourselves directly with the fluency problem, help should be given, at this early stage, with language development itself. Where a shock or some emotional disturbance, such as hospitalization or separation from the mother is given as the 'cause' of stuttering, there is a tendency to dismiss it, because it is felt that it could not be the sole cause. However, there is no doubt that trauma is in some cases contributive, at a stage when speech is vulnerable to disruption, and it could be that insufficient attention is paid to these experiences. If the emotional aspect were treated early enough, it is possible that the speech symptoms could be alleviated before they have become more complex through the contribution of reaction and the establishment of abnormal speech patterns. By the time a more advanced stutter has developed, the original trauma may well have become irrelevant.

Many children, of course, develop language quite normally to the almost adult level of the five-year-old before disfluency occurs and there is no report of shock or disturbance. We have little understanding of the causes of disruption here, except that some of them appear to come with the onset of schooling. Whether emotional pressures in a new environment are truly the direct cause of the difficulty we cannot say, with so little data at our disposal. One fruitful line of investigation could well be into the many factors which play a part in the child's experience of this period of change. We would need to have some understanding of the previous and still present environment of home, to consider the physiological and emotional demands made on these children and the role of cognitive and sociolinguistic development at this stage, all of which might throw some light on the breakdown in their speech, when faced with the need for adjustment. Again, such investigation should be made right at the onset rather than later, when behaviour has already become modified by the fact of stuttering itself.

Much more needs to be known, too, about the reaction to stuttering at this stage. Parental counselling is based on certain assumptions concerning those reactions which precipitate and perpetuate stuttering and others which will mitigate the problem. Some of this is common sense, and the withdrawal of 'adverse' reactions, such as over-anxiety or correction, will often result in the child's improvement. But, as far as we know, no thorough study has ever been made of different patterns of behaviour towards the stuttering child. Johnson's investigation into the onset of stuttering (1959) covers a good deal of ground, but he contrasts the responses of parents of stuttering children with those of parents whose children showed only normal nonfluency, rather than comparing differing approaches by parents whose children have begun to stutter. Such a comparison would help us to understand the problem of cases in which parents seem to approach the child in the ways advocated and yet still he continues to stutter. If we knew more, too, about the reactions of others in the child's environment—his peers, his teachers —we might know better where and how to modify them, especially linguistically, and prevent their contributing to attitudes towards communication which will perhaps become the greatest stumbling-block in his attempts to overcome the problem in the future.

Despite the impressive work of writers such as Bloodstein and Van Riper (see chapter 6), our knowledge of the development of stuttering from early disfluency to advanced stuttering in all its complexity is lacking in detail.[1] Van Riper's four tracks (chapter 6, pp 87-8) hold a valuable approach to the problem, but the lack of substantial longitudinal data prevents their being any more than this. We all believe that certain factors outside and within the child contribute to the growth of both overt and covert symptoms, to the development of inappropriate attitudes and to the buildup of a set of personal constructs deeply influenced by stuttering; but until all these elements have been sensitively traced in a far greater number of cases than Van Riper was able to study, there is little hope of our having enough information on which to base effective preventive measures. The detailed case-records required are time-consuming and would demand facilities and staffing which are far beyond our means, in the UK at least. However, more could be done even now if the importance of such work were recognized and more resources allocated in the direction of research aimed at contributing to greater understanding of the problems involved and therefore more effective treatment. Therapists in Britain tend to work too much in isolation. With a centralized policy, it should be possible for this sort of developmental data to be gathered and pooled at not too great a cost.

Without more detailed knowledge of the development of stuttering, we are inevitably working in the dark to a great extent in our treatment of adult as well as childhood disfluency. We suggested in chapter 6 an outline for a thorough assessment of advanced stuttering, but we are by no means happy that it is fully adequate. Such an assessment should give us some indication of the main needs of a particular speaker in the balance of work on the symptoms themselves and the psychological and environmental context in which they are manifested, but we are not satisfied that the picture is clear enough for appropriate measures to be taken in respect of every aspect of the problem. Though we may analyse in detail the overt symptoms, form a fair idea of the speaker's attitudes towards communication, his disfluency and himself as a whole, assessment of performance and emotional involvement in situations outside therapy is at present far from satisfactory. Once again, the technical facilities to improve this aspect and the personnel needed are not available. Yet, as with the accumulation of relevant developmental data, more could be done towards the establishment of better assessment procedures if therapists working in different centres could pool their resources to work together in an integrated and coherent way. At present, treatment results cannot be compared, as the tools for evaluation vary so widely.

Some research is currently in progress at the Speech Therapy Unit of the City Literary Institute, the main aim of which is to evolve an adequate assessment which will enable us to predict more clearly the responses of individual stutterers to different types and aspects of treatment. The project is too small and the facilities too slight to hope to show more than trends on which to base future work, but we feel that without some such attempt to evaluate our therapeutic techniques and those of others working in the field, we can only continue blindly trying this or

---

[1] Our knowledge of normal linguistic development is also far from complete and needs further investigation along the lines suggested in recent articles in the *Journal of Child Language*.

that measure and approach, with a confusion of success, partial success and failure as a result.

At present the treatment of stuttering is inadequate, mainly due to the lack of research already discussed and the failure of those attempting therapy to relate their work with one another and use more fully the resources of other disciplines. In one centre in Britain, a therapist with absolute conviction in the efficacy of a particular technique presents it to every stutterer, regardless of the nature of his problem. In some cases, of course, improvement is shown. Often it seems to be just that conviction which has the desired effect. At another clinic, a therapist with a more 'open mind' will try one technique after another with the same client, hoping to hit on something that will 'work'. Neither method is satisfactory and results are inevitably poor. Most therapists these days attempt to 'treat' the stutterer's attitudes, although the means of discovering these in any depth are not generally applied. Often the result is that the disfluent speakers become more confident and feel less afraid of tackling certain situations, but the therapists do not really know why, so that it is not possible to approach this aspect of treatment with more assurance. There is always the chance that an encouraging and perceptive friend could do as much or a change of circumstances produce a similar result.

Working in groups has come to be regarded as almost essential to the treatment of stuttering for many therapists. Stutterers themselves have expressed their feeling that the support of other members and the concerted efforts of a number of them give them encouragement that they do not find in individual therapy. No one, however, has researched into the factors which seem to make group work beneficial for many. We do not know which aspects of grouping produce the apparent motivation to continue the difficult work involved. Nor do we know for a fact that the effects of working in groups actually produce better results in the vital follow-up period, rather than simply making a particular course more stimulating at the time. In children's groups, such as those held at Blackfriars in London, some young stutterers are undoubtedly being prevented from developing avoidance reactions by having to go out to face difficult situations with their peers. At the City Literary Institute, the therapists believe very strongly in group work for many adults, for reasons both of the scope of material made available by numbers and the possibilities of understanding individual problems within the context of group discussion. But they have, as yet, no proof of their and their clients' beliefs, and it is certain that not everyone who comes to them is suited to this approach. Many who are, especially the more severe stutterers, clearly need individual attention as well; and some gain nothing, as they are not able to work in company with others. Investigation is long overdue into the efficacy of group speech therapy and it would surely be possible to find some measure of the suitability of particular people for this kind of setting.

In the United States there is a long tradition of research and experiment in stuttering therapy. Many of the universities have speech and hearing clinics with facilities for extensive programmes of treatment and the careful evaluation of those programmes. At the Speech and Hearing Clinic of Western Michigan University, for example, Van Riper and his colleagues have worked from 1936 to the present time, evolving new methods and continually reassessing their outcome. Clinical facilities at the University of California, Los Angeles, have allowed Sheehan to develop his 'role therapy' (1970, 260–310) after a long period of experimentation. Over several years, Ryan and Van Kirk (1974) have developed their programmed therapy for stuttering at the Easter Seal Rehabilitation Center and then the Behavioral Sciences Institute in Monterey, California. These are just a few of the many clinics and centres providing such opportunities for research and therapy.

Our comments on the treatment available for stuttering in Britain may seem so far very negative. However, despite the difficulties therapists face and the inadequacies of some of the work done, the situation is not hopeless. There seems to be a genuine move towards joint discussion and integration in the field of stuttering therapy, with the development of courses for therapists in centres specializing in the disorder. Greater links are being formed with other disciplines in an attempt to understand the problems more deeply, and experimental programmes such as that instituted at the Middlesex Hospital in London, with psychologists and therapists working together, are a healthy sign. Adult stutterers at least are no longer treated as 'patients', who are being offered a 'cure', but as colleagues in the search for control over a phenomenon which we need their help to understand. But a great deal more could be done. It should not be impossible to centralize our efforts and pool whatever resources there are for research into an integrated programme which could give us some of the information vital to us and to our clients. The following proposals may seem ambitious, but unless we plan for the future, no advances will ever be made in this area.

Some kind of central establishment is needed, not to dictate therapeutic methods, but to contain the data on the onset and development of stuttering discussed earlier. It should be a research centre, with contributions from many disciplines, so that various aspects of the disorders can be studied thoroughly and in a related and coherent way. Facilities for further investigation of the neurological and psychological aspects of speech production should be available. Articulatory aspects of speech production could be studied, using techniques such as cinefluography and electropalatography (see Hardcastle 1972). Laryngeal function can be examined by means of fibre-optic laryngoscopy (see Williams, Farquharson and Anthony 1975), electromyography (Tatham 1973), laryngography (Fourcin and Abberton 1971) and other similar techniques. And information concerning aerodynamic aspects of speech production can be obtained by means of oral and subglottal air-pressure records, electro-aerometry and spirometry. Information from these various sources will allow us to build up a more complete picture of the stuttering event itself as it occurs. For example, we may find that the location of stuttering is not necessarily related to linguistic factors, such as particular phonemes or parts of speech, but to a specific combination of articulatory, laryngeal and respiratory conditions. This complex of conditions may act as a trigger to the moment of stuttering. Also the possible involvement of sensory feedback mechanisms in both normal and disfluent speech should be investigated more fully, perhaps using recent experimental techniques such as anaesthetization of sensory nerves in the oral region (see for example

Gammon *et al.* 1971, Horii *et al.* 1973, Hardcastle 1975). This information would be important in testing the effects of such measures as masking, DAF or electromyographic feedback (see Guitar 1975) on individual stutterers.

It should be a centre where stutterers can attend for full and comprehensive diagnosis and where treatment is available to suit the needs of particular individuals. This would entail provision of many different types of treatment, but its administration would not be haphazard, as it so often is at present. Psychiatric help should be there for those who need it, techniques of control found to relate to a particular pattern of stuttering. And for some construct therapy should be available, where there is need to re-evaluate themselves and their world in relation to their speech (Fransella 1972). Individual therapy would play a large part for many, and group work, once its nature had been studied, would undoubtedly have something to offer most.

Research needs in cluttering

Much of what has been said in relation to further work needed on stuttering will, of course, apply to cluttering and perhaps the two should not be generally separated. However, since we have acknowledged its existence as a distinct type of disfluency, the greatest need here would seem to be to look further at the nature and origin of its characteristic manifestations. Basic phonetic studies in particular are needed. We should know more about the dynamics of articulatory behaviour in cluttering, with specific reference to the following: (*a*) Which segments and syllables are typically omitted? Are they the same as in normal fast speech? (*b*) Is the rate of articulatory movement itself greater for clutterers than for normal speakers, or is the well-documented increase in rate due primarily to shorter pauses? (*c*) Do the tonic stressed syllables remain relatively intact in cluttering, as they tend to in fast normal speech?

Clearly, an extension of the neurological investigations so far undertaken is indicated. The implications of the studies of Luchsinger and Landholt (1951) and Langová and Morávek (1964) (see chapter 8) cannot be ignored, and any further discovery as to an organic factor would advance our knowledge not only of the 'pure clutterer', but also the stutterer with cluttering as the basis of his disorder. Many questions remain unanswered here. In the earlier study, 90 per cent of the clutterers were said to have abnormal EEGs, in the second, 50 per cent—and so did some stutterers. It would be interesting to see whether a percentage of normally fluent speakers also showed these abnormalities. Were a further investigation to be made along these lines, other differences between the two groups—those who show EEG anomalies and those who do not—should also be studied. Is there any relationship, for instance, between the presence of other difficulties, with reading and writing for example, in the first group? The fact that a high percentage of clutterers responded well to the tranquillizing drug chlorpromazine suggests another fruitful line of work.

We have rather dismissed Weiss's over-generalizations about the personality characteristics and general language difficulties of clutterers, but nevertheless, where these other problems do exist, they should be acknowledged and studied more fully. It could be that, as with stuttering, we have subgroups of clutterers who should be distinguished from one another before treatment is planned. We suggested in chapter 8 that clutterers should be compared with those whose speech is rapid, though fluent, rather than continually contrasted with stutterers. Clutterers who show the hyperactivity and fast general movement which we have sometimes noted may in fact belong to a group otherwise considered 'normal', who also show these characteristics, but whose speech is not so noticeably affected.

The familial setting of clutterers has not been studied fully enough. Weiss claimed that most of his clients came from backgrounds whose speech and other language abilities were poor. Children 'at risk', in a family of fast, indistinct speakers could perhaps be taught more stable patterns of speech from the beginning. A number of our 'stuttering-clutterers' have spoken of fast-speaking, voluble parents, with whom they have always had to compete at home. Preventive measures could perhaps have been taken if this had been discovered early enough. We noted that many of our Asian clients seemed to have cluttered rather than stuttered patterns of speech. Some investigation into the nature of their original languages might prove useful in our approach to their particular problems.

In our discussion of the treatment of cluttering, we pointed out that although the needs are apparently less complex than those of much stuttering, the results are often as unsatisfactory. The difficulty so many of them experience outside the clinical situation in monitoring their output would seem to be the main problem. The slower rate needed for clear articulation is impossible for many of them to maintain, and better means need to be devised for establishing this altered pattern. Some kind of feedback system, signalling to them that they are increasing rate, might perhaps be helpful, if they could tolerate its use over a period long enough to allow for real change to take place. If it has been found possible to indicate to stutterers that muscle activity is increasing (Guitar 1975) or even to teach those with tachycardia to decrease their heart-rate (see Calder 1970) it would not be difficult to produce some sort of pace-setting instrument for clutterers.

Further research into the dysarthrias

The dysarthrias have been extensively studied, especially by such authors as Darley, Aronson and Brown (1969a, 1969b, 1975). In their work they discuss differential diagnostic patterns of the various types outlined in chapter 7, and they relate the clusters of deviant speech dimensions found in each type to their probable neuromuscular bases. They express the hope that their findings 'may serve as hypotheses for more accurate physiologic and neuro-physiologic measurements to further delineate the problems of dysarthria' (1969b, 462). We see the need for more objective techniques in studying aspects of the dysarthrias, rather than the largely impressionistic methods used by previous investigators. Some of the wide range of suitable electronic equipment at present available to study various aspects of speech production have already been discussed. Our hope is that such work will lead to some clear implications for treatment, since so far what we have to offer has severe limitations. We suggested in chapter 8 that our aims in therapy rested on the possibilities of strengthening muscle movement and control and developing careful self-monitoring in the speaker. This, as far as it goes, can lead to improvement, but there is great need for more knowledge and new techniques.

We mentioned in chapter 8 the use of brushing and icing to facilitate contraction of muscles (Draper 1968) and it is probably to physiotherapy that we must look for further development along these and other lines. There is some hope, too, in the progress made in drug therapy, especially in some cases of Parkinson's disease, where levodopa and its derivatives have proved effective for some aspects of the disorder (see Parkes and Marsden 1973). But until some chemical or other aid is produced that can repair or replace lost neural function, it is doubtful whether we can progress much further in our treatment of the muscular weakness and incoordination which is the basis of the problem in the dysarthrias. Research into brain mechanisms and their impairment is clearly of the greatest importance, and our present efforts without further knowledge are bound to be somewhat superficial and inadequate.

Further research into articulatory dyspraxia

We noted in chapter 8 that the very nature of the disfluency commonly called articulatory dyspraxia was in dispute. Not all the authorities are happy with the term itself, with its implications of a purely motor disability. The greatest lack, therefore, in this area would seem to be of a sensitive assessment of this kind of articulatory difficulty. We need to know not only the pattern of misarticulation produced by a particular speaker but, as we suggested earlier, the type of cue which will enable him to find the placement he requires, whether it be a strong visual stimulus for imitation, or an audible cue which appears to release a sequence of movements for him without direct effort. Nor should the dyspraxic element ever be evaluated in isolation from other aphasic difficulties. Evidence of impaired memory span, for instance, should be related to problems of retaining and reproducing sequences of phonemes. The speaker who has difficulty selecting from a flood of words which come to mind when he wishes to name something will probably also be flooded with alternative phonemes when he tries to initiate a particular word; while one who faces a blank in naming will face a similar blank when he searches for the position with which to start a word. In the first we may observe much struggle and retrial; in the second, no attempt until a cue is given. The patient showing the 'recurrent utterance' of a word or phrase at every attempt to speak, so often found in dyspraxia, is in yet another situation. His articulators move automatically into a set pattern, so that he has neither too much nor too little choice—the choice is made for him, rather like a gramophone needle stuck in a particular groove.

Until we are able to study such phenomena more systematically, planning therapy for the dyspraxic speaker will continue to be a hit-or-miss affair. We do not, as yet, know why associative work as suggested by Schuell et al. (1964) is effective for one, while Luria's articulatory diagrams (1970) appear to help another to restore his phonemic system. With some subjects, careful and laborious work on visual stimulation seems to be the only answer, but with others this method only leads to further confusion. The task continuum of Rosenbek *et al.* (1973) described in chapter 8, seems to hold the right approach in its step-by-step programming, but the results with the four subjects used were variable. No links were made with their difficulties at different stages of the task and the type of dyspraxic disorder shown by each in the context of the rest of their aphasic impairment. Much might have been learned from such a study. It could be frutiful not only to work on a refined continuum such as this, but also to note differences in response from a number of patients in relation to their language disabilities as a whole and the nature of their dyspraxia in particular.

Conclusions

It might seem from even such a brief survey of the inadequacies of our knowledge of disorders of fluency that attempts at remediation are likely to fail. But this is by no means the case. Many people who stutter, clutter or suffer from dysarthria and dyspraxia are greatly helped by the work of speech therapists and others concerned with their difficulties. Some have achieved a level of communication through treatment that they had not believed possible; others have reacquired speech skills, so that their lives could again encompass this especially human source of satisfaction. We cannot afford to rest, however, on the success accomplished. Those of us working with speech problems cannot be satisfied while so many aspects of the disorders remain a mystery to us and while so many of those who suffer from them remain beyond our scope. We cannot be daunted by the vast amount of research which still needs to be done or even by the lack of means to do it. If we set ourselves to relate more fully the work that can be done, it should be possible to advance our knowledge and thus our contribution to the treatment of disorders of fluency.

10

Developments in the understanding of stuttering and cluttering

Recent findings as to the nature and causes of stuttering

In chapter 5 an overview has been given of the main theories developed over the years as to the nature and causes of stuttering. We saw how at various times organic, psychogenic and 'learned behaviour' theories held sway. Today, although no-one doubts the importance of psychological, evaluative or environmental factors in the development of stuttering from its early manifestations, more weight is given to the likelihood of some degree of organic involvement at the very outset.

We described earlier (pp. 64–65) the research into auditory feedback and, in particular, Van Riper's proposal that a distortion in the total feedback system may be responsible for disfluency. Since then, developments in neuropsychological investigation have added credence, though by no means certainty, to some such theory of anomalous cerebral functioning. In an important recent publication (Rustin, Purser and Rowley 1987), Andrews hypothesises that 'due to an inherited or acquired deficit in their central cortical capacity for speech, stutterers have a diminished ability to deal with the relationship between motor activity and the associated sensory activity produced during speech' (xix).

In the same volume Rosenfield and Nudelbaum suggest more tentatively that some stutterers may well experience a breakdown of co-ordinated speech-motor output due to a disturbance in cerebral laterality, laryngeal motor control or the processing of signals. Moore and Boberg (31) find 'compelling evidence' from many studies that there are differences in CNS functioning amongst stutterers and favour the notion that greater right hemisphere processing may be the major difference. All agree, however, that no one neuropsychological factor has been found to distinguish the individual stutterer from the individual fluent speaker. There has been no suggestion that the presence of anomalies of CNS functioning makes treatment less viable. It would seem important never the less that where they are known their effects on speech production are taken into account when choosing the form of treatment to be undergone.

It also remains clear that although personality traits and environmental factors play an important part in what any particular disfluent person makes of his or her problem, there are no specific attributes or circumstances that can be said, in themselves, to contribute to the onset of the disorder. No-one seems to have followed up Van Riper's work in attempting to categorise stuttering into types or tracks according to features of onset and development (see pp. 88 – 99) and until more detailed and refined assessment becomes standard, such grouping is unlikely to be possible.

The origins of cluttering

In chapter 8 the etiology of cluttering was discussed. Although, again, no hard evidence was found to link all instances of cluttering with neurological symptoms, there was general agreement as to the probable existence of organic factors. Little further attention has been paid to cluttering in the literature since then. But one interesting paper (Wolk 1986) presents a diagnostic case report of admirable thoroughness. She explored the use of Luria's Neuropsychological Investigation (Christensen 1974) and a dichotic consonant-vowel (CV) listening task to highlight the symptomology in an adult clutterer. Although one single case study cannot safely be generalised, such a careful in-depth study can contribute much to the development of more appropriate assessments as a whole.

Besides the Luria investigation and the dichotic listening task, Wolk's procedures included a description of communication behaviour in terms of rate, fluency, articulation, voice and language skills together with neuro-anatomical investigations comprising a general neurological examination, an EEG and a CT brain scan. The communication profile showed clear if mild deficits in all areas, the EEG suggested some moderate fronto-temporal dysfunction, while the CT scan was normal. Luria's neuropsychological investigation showed up a slight disturbance in motor functions of the hand and a disturbance in acousticomotor organisation. It further highlighted the mild difficulties in expressing logical sequence of thought and the excessive repetitions and slight reading problem and pointed to slightly inadequate auditory memory span and sequencing skills.

With regard to the dichotic CV listening task, Wolk suggests that the client's overall ability in processing dichotic stimuli 'may indicate an "over-loading" to this clutterer's auditory system and may also reflect a generally lowered central auditory performance' (205).

Relatively slight as most of these findings are, they seem of potentially great importance with regard to the planning of therapy. Prognosis for cluttering is notoriously poor and Wolk suggests that one factor might be that insufficient attention has been paid to central auditory processing in these clients. She urges further research into such deficits with appropriate therapeutic goals in mind, such as an emphasis on increasing conscious attention, self-monitoring and tasks to improve auditory skills. Interestingly, her proposal that clutterers may need to be taught a volitional control over their entire speech output with the focus on language formulation, central auditory processing, articulation and prosodic features takes us right back to the general linguistic emphasis in the approach of Weiss (1966), based as they were on his sense of an 'organic flavour' to cluttering which at that time he was unable to substantiate. (Further aspects of therapy for those who clutter will be discussed later.)

Issues in disfluency assessment: early diagnosis

In Part One a detailed study of the speech variables involved in the evaluation of fluency is presented together with advances in linguistic profiling of stuttering. In chapter 6 the normal patterns of fluency development in children is traced and various views as to causes of disruption are considered. Later writers have continued to emphasise the difficulties involved in determining absolute definitions of stuttering as distinct from 'normal non-fluency'. Bloodstein (pp. 83–85) and Van Riper (pp. 86–89) as we saw give similar descriptions of early stuttering behaviour. Conture and Caruso (1987) in their review of various later attempts at measuring disfluency see Riley's Stuttering Severity Instrument and the Stuttering Prediction Instrument (Riley and Riley 1982) as 'important landmarks' in the field of stuttering in young people' (90).

One crucial issue related to the assessment of disfluency is the variability of stuttering discussed in chapter 4. Adults, as we have shown, may range from total fluency in one situation to severe blocking in another. With young children, these swings are even more marked with sometimes long periods of remission, lasting for days or even weeks. If a parent brings a child to the clinic during a fluent period the therapist may have nothing to go on but the parent's description of remembered behaviour, the contexts and so on. In this instance, it is useful to ask the parents to record their child's speech in a variety of situations over a period of time.

There is now more general agreement on the need for thorough assessment of many aspects of communication besides the disfluency itself. We noted in chapter 6 that Andrews and Harris (1964) and Morley (1957) found significant evidence of speech delay and articulatory defect amongst disfluent children and in later studies Riley and Riley (1979, 1983) list attending disorders, auditory processing disorders, sentence formulation disorders and oral motor disorders as occuring frequently amongst a sample of children screened. These difficulties should clearly form part of the treatment programme for such children. Conture and Caruso routinely assess receptive and expressive language, articulation, neuro-motor (non) speech behaviour, voice and reading skills along with the disfluency itself.

Assessing disfluency in older children and adults

In Part One and chapter 7 we discuss the complexity involved in assessing confirmed stuttering. We consider the issues of what to assess and when and apart from our own profiling, present details of two approaches to rating speech behaviour in the clinic (pp. 105–106), that of Johnson, Darley and Spriesterbach (1963), meticulous and exhaustive in its detail and that of Andrews and Harris (1964), far simpler. Perkins (1981) questions the usefulness of the Iowa Scale (Johnson et al) as not distinguishing between normal non-fluency and stuttering. He sees the measurement of 'syllable disfluencies per minute' as the most appropriate and convenient for clinical use. Although information is lost here as to types of disfluency, these can be noted alongside the percentage and the presence of prolongations, for example, or multiple repetitions will be shown up in loss of rate.

Hayhow (1983) addresses the question of what might be a representative speech sample, given the variability of stuttering referred to earlier. She considers counting syllables versus 'phone rate' in terms of accuracy and summarises current arguments regarding the measurement of concommitent behaviours. She emphasises the importance of assessing the stutterer's *fluent* speech, referring to Adams and Runyan's concept of 'tenuous fluency' (1981). This was found to be characterised by slowness, dysrythmia, weakness, tension, tremorousness and imprecision in articulation. Noted particularly in the speech of those who stutter more severely, Hayhow believes it to be an important dimension in over-all assessment which 'may well prove to have prognostic implications' (28).

Far more controversial than any views on assessment of speech behaviour remain those on measurement of attitude and self-concept, which we shall consider in a later section.

Stuttering in context: environmental factors

With regard to children, Conture and Caruso (1987) stress the importance of the information gained from parental interview, since they see stuttering as related to the interaction between not only fluency and other skills and abilities in the child but also between these and factors in the environment. Although this view has long been held by workers in the field, this aspect of assessment has become more comprehensive. Rustin and Cook (1983) for example, outline a very detailed procedure, aimed at evaluating family systems and structure, which should not only throw light on the child's situation but will ascertain 'the degree to which parents are able to participate in therapy without disturbing their equilibrium' (53) — a crucial issue when planning work with children.

Hayhow and Levy (1989) working from a personal construct perspective (which will be discussed in more detail later) see understanding the family as essential to effective therapy with children. They explore the background through the family tree or genogram and consider the family life cycle through which each member is passing. They look at the family construct system within which parents and children interact and believe that observation of this interaction and the communication between family members provides essential knowledge for the therapist.

Although school assessment is generally seen as important for the older child, rather less attention has been paid to nursery or play-school as part of the young child's environment. As a number of children experience their first awareness and frustration in relation to starting, say, at play-group, the reactions of teachers and children outside the family should be taken into account. Thompson (1983) includes assessment of teachers' handling of the disfluent child in their Assessment of School-Age Children, which would seem to provide a useful basis for dialogue with those involved with children at risk at this early stage. Cooper (1987) also includes a 'Teacher Assessment Inventory' in his battery. An infant teacher or play-group leader in a position to compare the speech skills of a number of children can be the first to draw the parents' attention to the difficulty which may initially occur in an environment where there is more pressure on speech than at home.

However, with the very young child, response to questionnaires about the child's behaviour does not seem to us to be enough. Careful exploration between therapist and teacher or play-group leader can sometimes bring out points of observation on the latter's part that might not be included in general questions, as they are special to the particular child. One infant teacher, for exmple, was the first to show concern about a boy's speech and general behaviour at school which was far less apparent at home. He not only produced disfluencies a great deal more severe than those heard by his family but had begun to use highly idiosyncratic devices to cover up his difficulty and get the attention he failed to do through words. He adopted strange postures, facial grimaces and emitted animal noises. These made the other children laugh sometimes, frightened them at others. He was fast becoming the class-room clown and it seemed that this role was the only one in which he felt effective. Fortunately the teacher made the connecton between his speech difficulty and his bizarre solution to it and referred him to speech therapy rather than any other agency. The effect of improvment in speech and confidence for this boy also produced advances in learning and peer relationships.

While factors in the environments of children and young people are generally investigated and taken into account, we find no evidence of any systematic exploration of the context in which the adult who stutters may be functioning. Their perceptions of specific speech situations have of course been explored by some workers such as Johnson, Darley and Spriesterbach (1963) with their 'Stutterers' Self-Ratings for Reactions to Speech Situations'. Fransella and others have also used Situations Grids to focus on this aspect. But an impression of the client's life-style as a whole: work involvement, home life, social activities, tends to be gained more informally through conversation over time. It would seem to us that knowledge of such factors as responsibilities, time pressures and the range of relationships encountered at work as well as the amount and kind of speech involved in a person's job is important from the outset. Time spent in activities with family and friends, responsibilities towards others and the degree to which the adult who stutters participates in conversation at home and socially can be significant. A person who lives alone, does a largely isolated job and seldom mixes with others will have different needs from one who is involved in family life, interacts frequently with colleagues at work and is active socially.

Although such a picture may emerge over time it can be useful to ask the client early on to make his or her own assessment of active involvement in situations, particularly those requiring speech during, say, a typical day at work and at home. One man who came for therapy and could only say vaguely that he 'didn't talk to people much' went away to note down his encounters on two such days. His report back was of three greetings first thing in the morning at work, one 'phone-call and two brief conversations with colleagues. Over lunch he spoke to no-one, although he sat with a group of people he had known for a long time. At home, where he lived with his parents, the very few exchanges with them during a Sunday were, he thought, typical. It was clear that any plans for work on fluency needed to include an appraisal of the implications for him of changes in interactions with others.

In contrast, a woman with considerable responsibility in her profession noted down:

Work Day: Numerous greetings first thing.

½ hour meeting with two colleagues (I probably did half the talking!).

Dictation to secretary: 20 minutes continuous speech.

¾ hour meeting with M.D.: fairly heated argument. Speech evenly divided.

Numerous short conversations including 3 'phone-calls.

Lunch: working lunch with colleagues. Again I did most of the talking.

½ hour of peace to begin the afternoon.

Disussion with colleagues led by me. Two of us did most of the talking.

2 or 3 'phone-calls, one lasting 20 minutes.

Mainly quiet for the rest of the afternoon (not typical).

Saturday   All talked at once over breakfast as usual.

Met one or two neighbours out shopping. Chatted briefly.

Lunch: Usual hub-bub.

pm. Children's friends to tea. *They* did most of the talking.

Eve: Dinner with friends. Dominating guest led to my being unusually quiet.

Long conversation with husband before sleep.

(MUCH HARDER TO JUDGE THAN WORK DAY)

Although this record served its intended purpose well, it proved a learning experience for the client in a number of ways. She had not realised that she talked so much. In observing the interactions at work she had noticed how much she interrupted others, how urgently she spoke and straight away questioned whether such urgency was part of the problem, causing extra pressure on her speech and leading to increased disfluency. Her reversal of behaviour in the face of the 'dominant guest' with the discomfort it involved also gave her pause for thought. 'Effective Communication', including listening skills became the primary goal for her which she elaborated more widely than her original aim for fluency.

Assessing people's everyday lives in this way can give client and therapist important information with regard to general pressures and demands as well as speech demands and involvement. Efforts at generalising fluency gained in the clinic to situations outside will often be dependent on some changes being made in order to reduce pressures or prepare for greater pressure which may come through greater involvement. More productive time and energy management can be a significant feature in improving communication for many adults.

The assessment of attitudes and self-concepts

In chapter 6 we discussed the importance of the child's attitudes towards stuttering as a part of our over-all assessment of the problem. And there remains no doubt in our minds as to the effect that confirmed negative attitudes may have as opposed to passing frustration at the time disfluency occurs. There *is* controversy, however, as to how these attitudes are measured and the validity of those measures (see below). Little is said of the origins of attitudes in the pre-school child and we know of no attempt to evaluate the signs of them. Because these are largely non-verbal it is probably not considered 'scientific' enough simply to observe and note them and include them in our plans for therapy. Cooper (1987), for example, simply says that his 'Attitudunal Indicators of Significance of Stuttering Checklist' is inappropriate when assessing the pre-school child. Nothing is suggested in its place. It does seem, though, that some means should be found to gauge the child's feelings around stuttering, without asking them the sort of question which would draw their attention to it too much. A therapist can make inferences from the child's behaviour when disfluent: flinching, colouring, excessive tension, loss of eye-contact, avoidance of specific words or becoming angry or silent, for example, will alert him or her to disfluency's being a negative experience for the child. Careful observation and checking out these inferences through further observations is essential here and should lead to appropriate guidelines as to how the child can be helped at these moments. Ignoring the signs can be the beginnings of the 'conspiracy of silence' experienced so painfully by many young children. It is from this, as well as from inappropriate negative reactions from others that more set 'attitudes' may grow. (See Dalton 1988 for examples of the use of behavioural observations in work with young children.)

There is no more scientific assessment of the development of attitudes towards speech difficulty in young children. Certain doubts are expressed as to reliability in using such procedures as Guitar and Peters' Nine Item A-Scale (1980) or Brutten's Speech Situations Checklist (1982) adapted for young people with older children. Some informal impression at least needs to be gained, however, since, as Cooper (1979) states, 'any stuttering program is inadequate if it does not at some time assist the individual in identifying and clarifying his feelings and attitudes about stuttering and fluency control' (85).

It is in relation to adults, however, that controversy about the assessment of attitudes has mainly persisted. As Hayhow (1983) states: 'There are some who believe that the problems involved in this area of investigation are so great that resources are better spent refining the assessment of observable and measurable behaviours'. Others continue to attempt the difficult task and such procedures continue to be in use. We discussed Erickson's 39-Item S-Scale in some detail in chapter 7 (pp. 108–110). Andrews and Cutler's modification in the form of the S-24 remains the most popular in use amongst clinicians despite the severe challenge in the journals by Ingham (1979). He believes that it has not been proven that the scale measures 'feelings about speech' as distinct from the person's perceptions of their 'speech behaviour' in certain situations.

In Dalton (1983) the issue of the importance of a wider view of the person who stutters than his perception of himself as a speaker was raised. Owen's contention (1981) was referred to as vividly expressing the point:

A specific behavioural adjustment takes place in a social context and within an individual life-style. We do not deal with addicts, alcoholics or stutterers, we deal with people whose lives are multifaceted and complex and whose specific behavioural disorder is part of a pattern of behaviour, thought processes, interpersonal relationships and environmental contingencies (59).

Being in total agreement with such a view we believe that perhaps the most important aspect of assessment is that of the child or adult's self-concepts, their views of themselves and their worlds. Sheehan (1979), Florance and Shames (1980) among others do express concern about the self-concepts of people who stutter but seem to limit that concern to their perceptions of themselves as communicators. The growing number of us who work within a personal construct theory frame-work (Kelly 1955), believe that knowledge of the person's perceptions of themselves as a whole, their main preoccupations and the major themes which govern their construing of events can help us to plan therapy which will be effective *for that particular person*. It should be stressed that the purpose of the exploratory procedures to be described is not to look for hidden weaknesses, skeletons in cupboards or deep psychological traumas but simply to try to know and understand the people we are working with in a deeper way.

There are by now many accounts of the personal construct approach within the literature on stuttering (Fransella 1972, Dalton 1983, Hayhow and Levy 1989, for example). We shall therefore present here a few of Kelly's main principles as they relate to the exploration of aspects of a person's way of construing. Kelly sees us all as attempting to make sense of ourselves and events through our systems of *personal constructs*, which we have developed throughout our lives from our experience of things and our interpretation of their meaning. Bi-polar constructs, such as 'pleasant ... unpleasant', 'gentle ... harsh', 'ambitious ... content with what they have' are the structural basis for these discriminations, the dimensions along which we make discriminations between people and events that occur. It is important to stress that construing is not the same as thinking. We construe with our eyes, ears, through touch and smell. Our emotions are inextricably linked with our thought-processes as we construe and behaviour itself is seen as part of our attempt to anticipate events in the light of how we have viewed them so far. Constructs are not the same as verbal labels — we need always to check what people mean by what they say. Many constructs cannot be verbalised. They may have been formed before a person developed language and remain largely inaccessible except through indefinable 'gut-reaction'.

The person creates an increasingly complex system of constructs as experience widens and although organised, this system is seen not as fixed but as capable of change through the modification of existing constructs, the creation of new ones and the discarding of old ones no longer useful. When we seek to explore with the child or adult client aspects of this system which make up his or her personality, we are attempting to see the world through their eyes and thus approach the problem in the context of an individual life-style as Owen suggests above. If they are to change as important an aspect of themselves as speech, the change must be compatible with the person who is changing, with what they might wish to become as a whole.

Since for many, unfortunately, personal construct psychology is 'about grids' and these are seen as inevitably complex, therapists have been slower to use the approach with children. However, not only have Repertory Grid Technique and Self-characterisations (to be discussed in more detail later) both been modified for use with children (see Salmon 1976, Ravenette 1975, Jackson and Bannister 1985) but the work of practitioners such as Ravenette (1977, 1980) has produced other simple and effective means of eliciting the construing of young people. With his 'Portrait Gallery' they may be asked, for example, when shown drawings of faces in varying moods 'What three things can you think of that make a person happy, sad, cross, frightened etc.' And they will usually tell you what makes *them* happy or sad. Ravenette's Self-evaluation procedure gets to the heart of a child's self-constructs when they are asked to say three things that each of the important people in their lives might say about them. One child had almost everyone describing him as 'worrying about things' and most of them also said that he 'wasn't very clever'. The basis of his poor self-image was clear. 'Troubles in School' are a set of deliberately undefined pictures which the child interprets as he or she sees them. In describing the scenes the children invariably present what are problems for *them*, what their solutions typically are.

These and many other procedures, some involving drawing, handling models or role-play are economical ways of coming to understand the child's ways of looking at things. Further examples of their use can be found in Dalton (1986, 1988) and Hayhow and Levy (1989). It is continually stressed that the therapist at no time imposes his or her views on the child, is, in Kelly's words, using the 'credulous approach', where the client's construing is accepted, his or her interpretation taken as their personal reality.

With older children and adults, Repertory Grid Technique and Self-characteristics are the most usual tools for exploration, although constructs can be elicited by a variety of means. As these procedures are now well-documented in recent literature on stuttering our discussion of them will be brief. A grid, for example, consisting as it does of a sample of the client's constructs obtained through comparing and contrasting significant people in their lives (the elements) will give us information about the content and the nature of a person's construing. We learn the important dimensions along which they make their discriminations, such as 'understanding ... insensitive', 'achiever ... failure'. We see where they place themselves and others on these constructs. And through computer analysis of grid data we learn something of the structure of their system: the tight construing shown by high construct relationships and the loose construing by low, for example, will imply different approaches for those with more set ideas about themselves and their worlds and those with, perhaps, more room for manoeuvre or even confused perceptions.

A grid which shows a large number of elements highly related on positive poles and the person himself or herself isolated in contrast on negative poles will suggest the need both for greater discrimination between others and reconstruction of the self in less depressive terms. The client may be asked to include specific self-elements such as Me Now as a Whole, Me Stuttering, Me as I'd Like to be, Me Fluent. The relationships between them can tell us how central their role as stutterer may be, how far they see fluency as taking them towards the self they wish to be and so on.

Botterill and Cook (1987) in the case study included in their chapter on personal construct work with adolescents analyse the young person's grid in some detail. Other examples of a variety of grids used with those who stutter can be found in Fransella (1972), Dalton (1983), Hayhow and Levy (1988). Fransella for instance described Situations Grids where speech situations are the elements instead of people.

Self-characterisations also furnish us with a picture of how the clients see themselves. They are asked to write a description of themselves in the third person as if through the eyes of an intimate and sympathetic friend. No guidelines are given as to content and the client's choice of themes and contexts can tell us much about what is important to them in their lives. Some write largely about their problem, others about relationships or work, others describe their lives historically, placing emphasis on events and people in their past. Whatever their perspective, it will help us to have some understanding of the person's view. Writing about themselves in the future or in the past can clarify for them what they might become or how they feel they have changed over time. (For a fuller discussion of this procedure see the texts named above.)

Summary of assessment issues

It will be seen from this section that assessment today in the view of many clinicians needs to be far more comprehensive than a decade ago. Some maintain that knowledge of brain functioning should be taken into account. In most clinical settings it would clearly not be possible to screen clients as thoroughly as we might wish, but perhaps selective neuropsychological screening should always be undertaken where there are signs of possible anomaly. Although, as we have said, there are those who believe only in measuring aspects of speech, others see careful exploration of the environment as essential and would not plan treatment without some understanding of the person, child or adult, with whom they are working. Simply putting a client through the therapist's favoured programme would seem, in any event, to be highly inappropriate.

While thorough assessment is clearly necessary for the purposes of planning treatment, its other function, as a basis for evaluating the effectiveness of therapy, is obviously of equal importance. Those who believe that the one criteria for success is the attainment of a specific level of fluency will focus their concern on this variable only. Others, who see the quality of that fluency as important will include measures of quality also. Still others who are interested in the effects of changes on the person as a whole will use procedures for appraisal of the people's views of themselves as a whole.

Recent advances in the treatment and management of stuttering: the controversies

In our sections on treatment in chapters 6 and 7 we touched on some of the broader issues with regard to planning therapy: how 'direct' work should be with young children (pp. 93–94), the differing aims of easier stuttering or total fluency with older children and adults (p. 114), questions of how the psychological aspects of the problem might be approached. In a significant book, published in 1979 Gregory invites a number of clinicians to address a range of 'controversies about stuttering therapy', which include but go beyond those mentioned above:

1. Teaching the stutterer to "stutter more fluently" versus teaching the stutterer to "speak more fluently"?
2. Attitude change: what is it and is it needed?
3. Psychotherapy for stutterers: what is it and is it needed?
4. The appropriate management of stuttering in children.
5. Planning the transfer of changes to the natural environment and dealing with the problem of relapse.
6. Criteria for assessing the results of stuttering therapy; reports on results of therapy (1).

Gregory himself contributes a review of thought about these questions and authors/clinicians with different orientations respond to them with, generally, highly reasoned arguments.

Those on the question of teaching the stutterer to "stutter more fluently" versus "speak more fluently" run along similar lines to our earlier discussion. We have addressed the issue of measuring attitudes and attitude change in our section on assessment. Some of these authors (eg. Ryan and Webster) not only see no need for the measurement of attitudes with the difficulties involved referred to above but maintain that work on attitudes is unnecessary since changes here automatically come about with changes in speech. Others, such as Perkins, Sheehan, Cooper and Williams, though not happy with current assessment procedures in this area do believe that attention to attitudes in therapy is important.

Some clinicians not only see a psychotherapeutic dimension to speech therapy as unwarranted but regard it as beyond the speech therapist's role. Williams, however, sees the speech therapist's role in this respect as having many links with that of psychotherapists and counsellors in other fields but maintains that our concern should be 'specific to speech and language problems'. Most see referral to a psychotherapist as necessary where a stutterer is found to have more complex psychological difficulties. Sheehan, for whom 'the relationship of psychotherapy to speech therapy and the degree of compatibility or co-existence of both behavioural and psychotherapeutic approaches' has long been of interest, believes that through his 'conflict theory' the two are 'potentially and logically compatible in conception, if not always practised' (192). His writings suggest that his major concern is with the psychological implications for the person as a communicator just as Williams implies. We believe that training in the personal construct approach to therapy should equip the speech therapist to fulfil the more comprehensive role needed.

With his questions about the transfer of changes to the environment, dealing with relapse and criteria for assessing the results of stuttering therapy Gregory opens a dialogue between clinicians which was to have far-reaching effects. As we shall see in a later section, maintenance of change has more recently become the most important focus of concern internationally.

Some developments in therapy for children

There are still differences in approach to stuttering in young children, mainly centred on the question of how much direct work should be undertaken with the disfluent child and how much through parental guidance. The shift in emphasis, however, has been towards an increase in both. There have been developments along the lines of more detailed 'programming'. Webster's Precision Fluency Shaping Program, for example, whose evolution is described in Webster (1980) has been modified for children. But although he believes that 'tight focus speech reconstruction therapy is particularly appropriate for young stutterers' he advocates using 'a light touch' and involving one of the parents for monitoring purposes. Cooper, too (1987) recommends 'an aggressive intervention approach with the very young child', based on a number of assumptions, including the belief that 'Very young children can be taught to use fluency initiating gestures efficiently and effectively' (131).

Rustin (1987) states that she has 'abandoned the notion that stuttering will simply go away if we ignore its development in young children' (166) and presents an approach to treatment combining direct intervention and active parental involvement. She cites a number of programmes for direct intervention, such as Cooper's and Shine's 'Systematic Fluency Training for Young Children' (1980) and describes the involvement of parents in counselling sessions, practice of speech techniques and cognitive problem-solving techniques as well as sessions where family management is considered.

Conture (1982) approaches therapy with young children very much with individual differences in mind. He describes those who are 'eager and ready' for speech therapy, 'quick studies', as opposed to those who 'hang back and appear to resist' or, when asked to leave their parents 'kick and scream as if being led to the gallows'. The management here will clearly need to be quite different in each case. Parents, he says, like their children 'come in all sizes and shapes and their idiosyncracies will influence therapeutic success' (41). Although such distinctions are implied in the careful assessments of children, parents and their family environments referred to earlier, this author in particular seems to have them in mind throughout his preparation for therapy.

He also considers issues involved for older children, such as motivation. Simple awareness of the fact that you stutter does not automatically bring with it the drive to work on the problem. Rustin and Purser (1984) discuss the social skills aspect of work with adolescents, who may miss out on this important dimension of learning because of their disfluency. Working in groups has been found to facilitate improvement in both these areas. In general, it can be seen that there is a move towards a broader perspective in many of the current approaches to work with young people.

Developments in therapy for adults

As with children, therapy for adults in the last decade has seen a move away from the simple choice of this or that technique as the 'right' one or this or that programme as 'the best'. While some clinicians continue to refine their particular programmes, others are more willing to offer choices according to the specific needs of the client. Cheasman (1983), in her overview of current techniques and programmes describes how at one specialist centre, the City Literary Institute in London, the first three days of the course are seen as largely diagnostic and, among other things, clients experiment with trial therapy procedures to see just how useful various approaches to fluency may be for them. The outcome decides whether they follow a Van Riper type of programme (stutter-more-fluently), described more fully in Reid (1987) or a slowed speech programme (speak-more-fluently), and within those programmes clients are encouraged to focus on the aspects most suitable for them. In individual treatment trial therapy can lead to an even more personalised approach to speech modification, agreed between client and therapist. It is important to stress that such a choice is made with care, not random eclecticism. Behavioural techniques may also change as the client changes and, throughout, joint evaluation of effectiveness is an essential part of therapy.

Developments in personal construct therapy with children and adults

Our brief reference to the work of Fransella (1972) in chapter 7 (pp. 118-9) gives little indication of the impact that Kelly's theory of personality (1955) was to have in the next ten years in Britain at least. In 1983 Dalton gave an account of some developments in the personal construct approach to stuttering. By then, her own and other's experiences led her to refute the earlier doubts as to the range of application expressed in chapter 7 (p. 118). Since then other accounts of such therapy have appeared, eg. Hayhow on work with children, Dalton on individual work with adults, Evesham on group therapy, all in Levy 1987. Botterill and Cook (1987) discuss their work with adolescents. And, recently Hayhow and Levy (1988) have produced the most comprehensive account so far, looking at work with children and their families, adults in individual therapy and in groups. As detailed descriptions of the personal construct approach are given in all the above texts, only a brief summary of its main aspects will be given here.

Attempts at reconstruction or personal change are based on the understanding of the person reached by client and therapist from the exploratory procedures referred to in an earlier section, from conversation and observation. This exploration itself, involving clarification and elaboration holds the beginnings of the reconstructive process for many and a relationship based on partnership is established. Where old ways of looking at the self and the world are found by both to be ineffective, experiments are set up to test out alternatives. The client may, for example, realise the need to develop greater understanding of others, attempting to see things through their eyes in order to relate to them more effectively. Situations in which they have been locked in patterns of construing which make their own part in them predictable but painful, may be approached in various ways until a looser repertoire for handling them is created. Aspects of the self may be equally trapped in unchallenged views. Having seen people as either 'aggressive' or 'holding back' and placed themselves on the latter pole as less threatening than the former, experiments in, say, 'quiet assertion' may lead them to reconsider their earlier construing.

Having less complex systems for construing, children are on the whole even more open to change if alternatives are found which have meaning for them. The development of a negative net-work of constructs around 'strangers' for example or 'teachers' due to some uncomfortable experiences can be arrested by active construing of strangers or teachers who are less threatening. The young boy mentioned earlier who saw himself labelled as 'worrying about things' was helped to highlight areas of greater confidence in himself while his mother was asked to validate other aspects of his approach to life besides his anxiety. A girl whose responses to the Troubles in School pictures was to get out of every situation through crying was willing to role-play other solutions and began to deal with events in a number of different ways.

Such experiments for change may be created through role-play, writing, drawing as well as conversation. Working in groups, clients learn to develop the credulous approach towards each other and can provide both ideas and encouragement. Such an approach to the psychological dimensions involved in no way precludes work on the speech itself. Dalton (1983) describes a group working within this framework in which members each had their own fluency aims, chosen in the light of their individual needs. Evesham and Fransella (1985) show from their research how two groups, one using the prolonged speech technique only, the other prolonged speech work combined with personal construct therapy compared in outcome. Progress in the latter group was significantly greater and better maintained than in the former.

Developments in the treatment of cluttering

In our earlier section on cluttering in this chapter we referred to Wolk's proposal that clutterers may need to be taught a volitional control over their entire speech output, with focus on language formulation, central auditory processing, articulation and prosodic features. Kelham (1978) in her account of therapy with a 6-year-old boy, began her work with him on the severe phonological disorder for which he was referred. Later, using language laboratory facilities, she focused on developing general language skills, with attention to reading and writing as well as speech.

From a different perspective, Marriner and Sansom-Fisher (1977) present a single-case study of an adult client where broader behaviour modification was attempted. Besides aiming to control speech rate, the programme included work on excessive 'dominance' in conversation and 'appropriate response to inter-ruption', pin-pointing two key aspects of this client's ineffective communication. Such attention to other aspects of personal interaction would seem to us very valuable on two counts. First, it places fluency in a broader spectrum of communication skills, especially important with a problem of cluttering. Second, it implies a two-way process, with those involved participating as listener as well as speaker. Sole emphasis on the 'performance' of the person who is disfluent seems to us to intensify the difficulty.

Our experience of working within a personal construct framework with those who clutter has shown this approach to be as relevant here. It emerged, for example, from the grid of an eleven-year-old boy that 'having something to be teased about . . . never teased' was a major dimension in his construing of people. Addressing this issue first and experimenting with alternative ways of dealing with teasing both eased this situation for him and increased his interest in working on speech. A young man had put all his difficulty in relationships down to other people's impatience with his unintelligible speech. It was clear, however, from his descriptions of people that he had little tolerance for their 'slowness' in every respect. Giving himself and others more time and space on a number of levels in his interactions proved to be of considerable value in the process of change.

It would seem from these few examples that there is a trend in the treatment of cluttering, too, to broaden perspective.

Evaluation of treatment and maintenance of change

Throughout the 1970s concern was growing at the apparent failure of various treatment programmes to bring about lasting change. There was ample proof that many approaches could lead to fluency within the clinical environment and the transfer of this fluency into life situations during the course and for a period of time afterwards. As more long-term follow-up assessments took place, however, the picture became rather bleak. In 1979 a conference was held in Canada which marked a turning-point in the history of therapy for stuttering (Boberg 1981). Here many of the issues to do with the evaluation of long-term outcome were addressed.

The familiar arguments as to exactly what should be measured and in what circumstances were reiterated. Whether or not the measurement of attitudes and self-concepts should be included was aired yet again. Doubts were cast as to the validity of most 'objective' measures and even greater ones with respect to self-report data. With the varying therapeutic approaches having different aims, how could we compare one set of criteria for success with another? And where does the person's own evaluation of his or her progress come in?

None of these problems was solved on this occasion but the focus on them was undoubtedly healthy. A number of ideas for maintenance work were exchanged. While most of the participants agreed that it was possible for many children to leave a period of stuttering behind them with appropriate management, the outcome for adults remained far more controversial. Approaches which aim at the elimination of disfluency would seem straight-forward enough to evaluate. But there are still questions as to what represents a reliable speech sample at a later stage. Reading, solo speech and conversation recorded within the clinic where treatment took place is clearly not evidence enough of the level of fluency in a person's daily life. Ingham advocated covert as well as overt measurement and over a period of time as the only reliable sample. (See also our discussion of Costello and Ingham (1985) in chapter 4 pp. 49-50.) Some, such as Perkins, regarded the quality of fluency as an important variable to evaluate and would include the speaker's own perception of its normalcy for him or her as part of that evaluation. Fluent speech which requires constant monitoring in order to be maintained was seen by him as just 'not cost-effective' (169) for most.

There was no-one amongst the speakers at the conference representative of the 'stutter-more-fluently' approaches where, presumably, measurement of changes in attitude and self-concept would be of equal importance to changes in speech. Although it is claimed by some that these aspects of change run parallel, work to ease anxiety, decrease fear and avoidance of stuttering, could result in greater psychological than behavioural changes in some. Personal construct therapy alongside speech modification procedures has shown this phenomenon in clients with mild disfluency but high anxiety.

Later studies on the effectiveness of treatment have continued to explore the many factors affecting outcome. St. Louis and Westbrook, for example, (1987) consider questions around the definition of success raised above, the general usefulness of various techniques and therapeutic models, variables amongst clinicians and clients. They present an impressive table of recent stuttering treatment studies, showing the growth of research in this area but their column giving 'Measure of Effectiveness and Averaged Results' (246-7) has little meaning since percentage gains in fluency over such varying lengths of time make any real comparisons impossible. There are no details as to how these measures are taken. They urge continuing 'thorough and relentless' self-examination by clinicians, while Purser, in the same volume, stresses the need for 'an increase in the amount of well-controlled comparitive outcome research' (273).

Hayhow and Levy (1988) address wider issues in their chapter entitled 'Continuing the Process of Change'. Their theory of relapse, based on personal construct theory, while acknowledging the many factors involved, presents the most obvious reason as that reversion to stuttering is the only pathway open to clients 'when the implications of fluency evoke anxiety, threat or guilt. When newly formed structures are invalidated, the person may abandon these in favour of previously used constructions (19). They see the need in later stages of therapy to focus on problems brought by clients which go beyond those directly related to speech itself: problems centred on the construing of the self as a whole, the construing of others and the threat that their experimentation in these areas might bring.

How far have we come?

The research needs into all the disorders of fluency outlined in chapter 9 over a decade ago still hold good to a large extent today. Psychoneurological and physiological investigation has advanced and will undoubtedly continue. There is evidence of greater interdisciplinary co-operaton such as we advocated and the specialisation of clinicians already established in the United States and elsewhere has developed in Britain over this period. As we have shown, evaluation of treatment had increased but its refinement is essential. Our dream of a central establishment for research and therapy has not become a reality. Therefore we must continue to share ideas through the literature, through conferences, through informal meetings and contacts until such time as these disorders are taken seriously enough to be regarded as worthy of the attention and resources they deserve.

Appendix

Phonetic transcription of disfluent speech

In the following two excerpts the speech of two disfluent speakers has been transcribed from a taperecording. Excerpt 1 is part of an interview between a severe stutterer (Speaker A) and a therapist (T). Excerpt 2 is a sample from Speaker B, a stutterer-clutterer. In each case an orthographic representation is included above the transcription. The phonetic symbols and main marking conventions used in the transcription are as follows:

Vowels		**Consonants**	
i	*as in* pit	p	*as in* pin
e	pet	t	tin
a	pat	k	kin
ʌ	putt	b	bay
ɔ	pot	d	day
u	put	g	gay
ə	potato		
		f	fin
iː	peat	v	vat
ɑː	part	s	sin
əː	pert	z	zoo
ɔː	port	ʃ	shin
uː	boot	ʒ	pleasure
		θ	thin
ei	bay	ð	that
ai	buy	h	hint
ɔi	boy		
au	how	m	met
əu	hoe	n	net
iə	pier	ŋ	hang
eə	pear		
uə	poor	tʃ	church
		dʒ	judge
		l	lip
		r	rip
		j	yet
		w	wet

Special diacritics and marking conventions

?	glottal stop
ₒ	devoicing (e.g. ḍ)
∿	creaky voice
ʰ	aspiration (e.g. tʰ)
→	prolongation of fricative or closure phase of stop consonant
ᴛ	increased muscular tension accompanying articulation
'	ejective release (e.g. t', s')
ˣ	affricated release of velar stop (kˣ)
ᶜ	lax palatal or post-alveolar click
…	breathy voice quality
ʷ	labialization
ˌ	syllabic consonant (e.g. ḷ)
*	brief pause
**	long pause
***	extra long pause (over 1 sec. duration) and end of utterance
|	tone-group boundary
ˈ	stressed syllable carrying relatively high pitch
ˌ	stressed syllable carrying relatively low pitch
ˋ	nuclear syllable of tone-group with high falling pitch
ˎ	with low falling pitch
ˊ	with high rising pitch
ˏ	with low rising pitch
ˇ	with fall-rise pattern
˃	with level pitch

Other symbols and diacritics used are those suggested in the International Phonetic Alphabet. In most cases the vowel sounds are transcribed using standard phoneme symbols, as there appeared to be few phonetically abnormal features in the articulation of these sounds by both speakers.

Excerpt 1

T and what is your job?

```
     I'm    an    ac-     ac-       count-    ant      in local
A   ˌaim ə̰ * ən ** ə̰ʔk *** ʔək *** ˋkˣaunt→*** tʰəntʰ ** | in ˈləukḷ ***

     government
     ˋg̊ʌvə ** məntʰ *** |
```

T oh, what does that cover?

```
     well   as you   as you  probab-           ly     know      we
A   ˋˋwəl * | aʒuː *** azjuː ˈpr̥ɔb→ *** b̊əb→** bliːʰ***ˊᵏnəu *** | wiː

     look after   the  roads  and      police     um housing
     ˈluk ˈɑːftə * ði ˀʰrəudz ənd *** | ˀᶜpl̥iːss ** | əm ˀhauziŋ ** |

     and these sort of
     ən ˋðiːz̥ sɔːt əv *** |
```

T and the rates and that kind of . . .

```
     yes   and um   we  just    look after  the um money     end
A   ˋjes * | ənd əm * ˈwiː ˈdʒəst→** ˈluk ˈɑːftʰə ðiəm ˋʰmʌniː * ˌʔend

     of it
     ʔɔv itʰ *** |
```

T yes . . .

```
     and I   personally         am an auditor         and we
A   ən ˈai ** ˅ᶜp̊əːsənʰliː | əb→** em en ˋɔːditʰə ** | ən ** ənd ˌwiːᵏ

     look after    the   things like   checking that all income has
     luk ˈɑːftə *** ðeə *** ˌθiŋz laiʔ ** ˌtʃekiŋ ʰðət ʔɔːl ˌʔiŋkʌm həz

     been  banked  and     you know this sort of
     biːn | ˌbaŋktʰ ənn ** | jə nəu ˋðis sɔːt əv *** |
```

T yes, do you have machines to help or don't you need them?

    oh yes   we   we use a lot of um   elec-
A ˈəu ˏjeə ** | wiːv * wiː ˈjuːz ˈļədəv ʌmm ** ʌm * ˈiːleʔkᶜ→ ***

    um elec-   tronic   aids
    əm ˈiːlek→*** ᶜᶜtrɔniʔk ˌʔeidʐ *** |

T like adding machines?

    yes and   elec-   um elec-   tronic
A ˋjes ən ʌm * | ˈiːleʔk→*** əm ˈiːleʔk→*** tr̥ ** ˈᶜtrɔniʔk *

       calculators
       tʰəˋkalʔk→*** kjuʰˌleitəz *** |

T oh, what are they?

    well that's   I mean whereas   one adds up   um if
A wel ˈˀðatss *** | ʔai miːn ˈweːrəz əˀ ** ᶜəzˈwʌn ˈadz ˋʌp *** | əm ˈif

    you want to   multiply   you'd have to have a
    ju ˈwɔntʰə ˇmʌltʰiʔp→*** pļai * | ˈjud ˈhav tə ˈhav eiː ***

    calculator
    ˋk̊ʰalkjəleitə *** |

T yes, yes, of course . . . where do you live?

    I live in um Bognor Regis
A ai ˈliv in ʌmm ˈbɒg̊nə ˏʰriːdʒis *** |

T have you always lived there?

    I've   been there most of my life   um but I have
A ˈaiv *** ˈbʌnə ðeə ˇməust * ʔɔv mai hˈlaif ** | əːm * bətʰ * ˈai ˈhʌg̊

lived   up in   up in   London   for one and a   a   um
** ˈᶜlivd ˈʔʌp ḭn *** ˈᶜʌp in ʰˠlʌn *** ᶜᵔᶜᵔ dən │ fə ˌwʌn ən ə * ʔei əm

half years   but I've   I've um moved   back
ˌhɑːf ˇjiəz ** │ bʌt ˌaiv ** ˌaiv əm ˌmuːvd̥ ** ˇᶜb̥akᶜᶜ *** │

about   six   years ago
ᶜbaut ** ˌs→iks ˋjiəz əˌgəu *** │

T   yes . . . where did you train?

at   well at   Chichester
A   ˈatʰ * wəl ˈat→*** ᶜᶜtʃitʃestə *** │

T   oh that's a nice place too . . . and do you have any hobbies?

yes   one   of   my   hobbies   is   music
A   ˋjeəs ** │ ˋwʌn * ˌɔf→** mai * ˌhɔb→*** biːz̥ * │ iz ˌmuːs→**ˋs'ik * │

and the other   one   is um   playing   hockey
ən ði ˇʌðə *** ˌwʌn │ iz ʌm ** ˌpl̥eiiŋ *** ˋhɔkiː *** │

T   when you say music do you mean do you like listening to it or do you play anything?

I   I actually   play in   two um   bands   and I
A   ˈai *** ai ˈaktʃəli *** ˋpl̥ei in *** │ ˌtuː əm ** ˋb̥andz̥ │ ˌən ˌai

also   like   listening   to   music
ˌɔls→*s'əu * ˌlaik ˋlis * ə * niŋ *** tʰuː ˈmuːs→* ˈs'ik *** │

T   what do you play?

I   um   well   my
A   aiʔ *** əmm ** wel *** ᶜmaiʰ ***

T I mean what instrument . . .

um   yes   quite   my   main   instrument   is the   um
A ˈmjeəːs │ ˈkwait *** │ ˌˤmai ˇmein ˈinstrə̩ ** mənt iz ði ** │ ʌm **

     is   the   bass   guitar   but I   also   play
ᶜhᶜhiz ði ʔ *** ˈb͡eis→* skwiː ʔ ** ˋtʰɑː *** │ bət ˈai ˈɔlsəuʰ ˈpl̥ei

        the um   banjo   and ordinary   guitar
*** ˈðum ˇban *** d ʒəu │ ən ˋɔːdinriː ** ˌgiː ʔ ** ˌtʰɑː *** │

Some general phonetic observations on the speech of A

1 Relatively frequent occurrence of pauses longer than 1 sec within tone-groups

2 Unusual distribution of pauses, many occurring, for example, within words (as in [ˈg͡ʌvə ** məntʰ])

3 Repetitions mainly of syllables, words and phrases

4 Frequent tensely articulated fricatives, stop closures and releases

5 Glottal-stop initiations of many vowels

6 Ejective release of some stops and fricatives (e.g. [muːs→ ** ˋsʼik])

7 Frequent use of preaspiration (e.g. [ʰrəudz] and [ʰmʌniː])

8 Abnormal prolongation of some fricatives (especially [s]) and some stop consonants (especially bilabials)

9 Relatively slow tempo

Excerpt 2

of of having a con-   just   of   having a conversation

B   ʔɔ ʔɔ ʔəvənə ˈkʰɔnf *** ˈdʒist ʔɔvəʔ * ɔv əvn̩ ə kʰɔnvəˋseiʃən *** |

um   as regards sport   as you know football   is in fact my main

əm * s̩ˈkɑːdz̥ ˇspɔːt * | ʃə   nə ˋfuʔtbɔl * | ˌiz in fakt mai ˌmein

sport   and I   am the manager   of a team   um   we're

ˌspɔːt ** | ən * ˈai ˈam ðə ˋmanədʒə *** | əy̥ ə ˋtʰiːm *** | ʌm ** wiə

not doing very well this season and   but the job that I do

nɔt ˈduːiŋ veri ˇwel ðis ˈsiːzn̩ ən ** | bət ði ˋdʒɔb ðət ai ˌdu * |

is mainly sort of   it's mainly sort of um   tearing about after

iz ˈmeinliː sədəv *** its ˈmeinliː sədəv əm * ˈtəːnn ˈb̥əut ʔɑː ʔɑːftə

players   and trying where to find players   for the majority of the

ˋpl̥eiəz * | ən ˈtr̥aiiŋ weə tə ˋfaind ˌpl̥eiəz ** | fə məˇdʒɔdʒi əfə

time   um looking after kit   the football kit

ˈtaim *** | əmʰ ˈlukən ɑːftə ˋkʰitʰ ** | ðə ˋfuʔbəl ˌkʰitʰ ** |

bit of first aid   if it is ever needed it if it is ever

bit əy̥ ˈfəːst ˋeid ** | ˈif it iz evə ˌniːdəd ət | if it iz evə

needed   very rarely happens though

ˌniːdəd *** | ˌveri reəliː ˌhapənz ðəu *** |

General observations on the speech of B

1 Relatively fast tempo

2 Frequent elision of syllables and sound segments (e.g. [s̩ˈkɑːdz̥])

3 Reduction of vowels

4 Some repetition of phrases, syllables and sound segments

5 Excessive coarticulation (e.g. [mədʒɔdʒi] = 'majority')

Linguistic profiling of stuttering

The following is a transcript of the first 100 words of Excerpt 1 (Speaker A) showing the coding used in the linguistic profiling procedure discussed in chapter 4 (based on Edwards and Hardcastle 1987).

Transcription conventions:

Tone group boundary: |

Nucleus of tone unit:
> the stressed syllable carrying the nuclear tone is in bold type e.g. **go**vernment

Syllable carrying rhythmical stress in the tone unit:
> ' placed before syllable e.g. "in 'local **go**vernment"

Type and location of a particular disfluency:
> Each disfluency is identified by a code consisting of an initial letter (referring to the tone group in which it occurs) a number (the temporal order in which it occurs in the tone group) and the type of disfluency (R = repetition, P = prolongation or PA = filled pause). In the transcription, the locations of elemental repetitions and prolongations are shown by underlining the element on which the disfluency occurs e.g. "'pro<u>ba</u>bly". Cluster, syllable, word, phrase and clause repetition are shown by repeating the relevant part of the target item in the transcription. Extra long pauses (i.e. those over 1 sec duration) which are perceived impressionistically as being unrelated to articulatory closures are indicated by an *. Filled pauses are indicated by an orthographic representation such as "um", "er", etc. The interviewer's utterances are written within brackets.

Transcript of Speaker A

(and what is your job)

    ⟨A1:R⟩ ⟨A2:R⟩ A3:P A4:P
A I'm an an   a - * a - **coun**<u>t</u>ant * |

        B1:P   B2:P
B in 'local **govern***ment |

(oh, what does that cover?)

C **well** |

D1:R   D2:P D3:P D4:P
D   as you * as you 'probably   **know** * |

E1:P
E   we'look 'after the **roads** and * |

F1:P
F   po**lice** |

G1:PA
G   um   **hous**ing |

H   and these sort of

(and the rates and that kind of)

I   **yes** |

J1:PA   J2:P   J3:PA J4:P
J   and um   'we 'just '**look**'after the um   **mon**ey 'end of it |

(yes)

K1:P K2:P
K   and I **per**son**al**ly |

L1:P L2:R
L   a**m**   am an **aud**itor * |

M1:R   M2:PA M3:P   M4:P
M   and *and 'we look 'after * the er * '**thing**s like '**check**ing that
all **in**come has been |

N1:P
N   **bank**ed and * |

O   you know **this** sort of |

(yes, do you have machines to help or don't you need them?)

P   oh **yes** * |

Q1:R   Q2:PA Q3:PA Q4:R Q5:PA   Q6:P
Q   we we   'use a lot of um * um   '**elec** um   'elec**tron**ic 'aids |

(like adding machines?)

       R1:PA

R   **yes** and um |

   (S1:R) S2:PA (S4:R)S5:P S6:R S7:P

S   'elec -um 'elec   tronic **calc**ulators |

(oh what are they?)

T   well **thats** * |

   U1:P   (U2:R)

U   I mean 'whereas as as 'one 'adds **up** * |

   V1:PA   V2:P

V   um   'if you 'want to **mul**tiply |

                          W1:P

W   'you'd 'have to 'have a **calc**ulator |

Symbols used in profiles

A	adverbial		O	object
Adj	adjectival		part	particle
Aux	auxiliary		Pr	preposition
c	coordinator		Pron	pronoun
C	complement		s	subordinator
cop	copular		S	subject
D	determiner		V	verb
Int	intensifier		osc	oscillations
Neg	negation		sub.cl.	subordinate clause
N	noun			

PROFILE OF STUTTERING BEHAVIOUR

Section 1 Repetitions

NAME: A
AGE: 38
DATE: 4-6-76
SAMPLE: CONVERSATION

TYPE	TARGET	REPETITION FREQUENCY (slow) 1	2	3	4	>4	LOCATION: PROSODIC LEVEL: HEAD + stress	HEAD − stress	NUCLEUS	TAIL + stress	TAIL − stress	WORD LEVEL: WORD INITIAL	WITHIN WORD	PHRASE LEVEL	CLAUSE LEVEL	TOTALS	
ELEMENTAL: STOP	/p/															/p/	
	/b/															/b/	
	/t/															/t/	
	/d/															/d/	
	/k/	S6							S6			S6		S6: DNPrAdj NcAdj N	S6: SVO	/k/	1
	/g/															/g/	
FRICATIVE	/f/															/f/	
	/v/															/v/	
	/θ/															/θ/	
	/ð/															/ð/	
	/s/															/s/	
	/z/															/z/	
	/ʃ/															/ʃ/	
	/ʒ/															/ʒ/	
	/h/															/h/	
AFF	/tʃ/															/tʃ/	
	/dʒ/															/dʒ/	
APPROXIMATE	/w/															/w/	
	/r/															/r/	
	/l/															/l/	
	/j/															/j/	
NASAL	/m/															/m/	
	/n/															/n/	
	/ŋ/															/ŋ/	
	VOWEL	(A2)						(A2)				(A2)		(A2): DN	(A2): SVCA	VOWEL	1
CLUSTER		(S4)						(S6)					(S6)	(S4): DNPrAdj NcAdj N	(S4): SVO	CLUSTER	1
SYLLABLE		(Q4) (S1)					(Q4) (S1)					(Q4) (S1)		(Q4): DNPrAdj NcAdj N (S1): DNPrAdj NcAdj N	(Q4): SVO (S1): SVO	SYLLABLE	2
WORD		(A1) (L3) (M1) Q1 (V1)						(A1) (L3) (M1) Q1 (V1)						(A1): DN (V1): sub (L3): cop (M1): S Q1: Pron	(A1): SVCA (V1) SVsub SVA (L3): cSAVC (M1): cSVO' Q1: SVO	WORD	5
PHRASE		(D1)						(D1)						(D1): c Pron	(D1): cSAV	PHRASE	1
CLAUSE																CLAUSE	
TOTALS		11					2	8	1			4	1			TOTALS	11

W. Hardcastle and S. Edwards, Department Linguistic Science, University of Reading

Fig. 9. Chart: Profile of stuttering behaviour, Section 1 Repetitions

PROFILE OF STUTTERING BEHAVIOUR
Section 2 Prolongations

NAME: A
AGE: 38
DATE: 4-8-76
SAMPLE: CONVERSATION

TYPE		TARGET	DURATION <1 sec.	DURATION >1 sec.	sec.	PROSODIC LEVEL: HEAD +stress	HEAD -stress	NUCLEUS	TAIL +stress	TAIL -stress	WORD LEVEL: WORD INITIAL	WITHIN WORD stable end	WITHIN WORD other	PHRASE LEVEL	CLAUSE LEVEL	TARGET	TOTALS
AUDIBLE	+ VOICE STOP CLOSURE	/b/	N1	D2 D3			D2 D3	N1			N1	D2 D3		D2: A D3: A N1: Aux Aux V	D2: c SAV D3: c SAV N1: c SVO'	/b/	3
		/d/														/d/	
		/g/		B1				B1			B1			B1: Pr Adj N	B1: SVCA	/g/	1
	- VOICE FRICATIVE	/f/														/f/	
		/θ/	M3			M3					M3			M3: DN Pr V	M3: c SVO'	/θ/	1
		/s/														/s/	
		/ʃ/														/ʃ/	
		/h/														/h/	
	+ VOICE FRICATIVE	/v/														/v/	
		/ð/		M3		M3					M3			M3: DN Pr V sub cl	M3: c SVO'	/ð/	1
		/z/														/z/	
		/ʒ/														/ʒ/	
	VOICE AFF	/dʒ/															
	APPROXIMATE	/w/														/w/	
		/r/	E1					E1			E1			E1: DN c NN c Adj N Pr	E1: SVO'	/r/	1
		/j/														/j/	
		/l/	J2 K2			J2				K2	J2	K2		J2: V part K2: A	J2: c SAVO K2: c SAVO	/l/	2
	NASAL	/m/	J4	B2 L1			L1	J4		B2	J4	B2	L1	B2: Pr Adj N J4: DAdjNPr Pron L1: cop	B2: SVCA J4: c SAVO L1: c SAVC	/m/	3
		/n/		D4				D4			D4			D4: V	D4: c SAV	/n/	1
		/ŋ/														/ŋ/	
	VOWEL															VOWEL	
SILENT	STOP CLOSURE	LAB		F1 K1 S7 V2			F1	X K1		V2 S7	F1 K1	V2 S7		F1: DN c NN c Adj N Pr K1: A V2: V V S7: DN Pr Adj N c Adj N	F1: SVO' K1: c SAVC S7: SVO	LAB	X4
		ALV	M4	Q6 A4 S5		M4	S5	Q6		A4	Q6 M4	A4 S5		Q6: DN Pr Adj N c Adj N A4: DN M4: DN Pr V sub. cl. S5: DN Pr Adj N c Adj N	Q6: SVO M4: c SVO' A4: SVCA S5: SVO	ALV	X4
		VEL		A3 W1				A3 W1			W1	A3		A3: DN W1: DN	A3: SVCA W1: A' SVO	VEL	2
	OTHER			U1			U1				U1			U1: Pron	U1: SVA'	OTHER	1
TOTALS			X 7	X 17		X 4	X6	X9		X5	X14	X9	1			TOTALS	X 24

W. Hardcastle and S. Edwards, Department Linguistic Science, University of Reading

Fig. 10. Chart: Profile of stuttering behaviour, Section 2 Prolongations

NAME: A
AGE: 38
DATE: 4-8-76
SAMPLE: CONVERSATION

PROFILE OF STUTTERING BEHAVIOUR

Section 3 Pauses

TYPE		LOCATION							
		Prosodic Level					Phrase Level	Clause Level	
Filled	Unfilled	Head	Nucleus Pre	Nucleus Post	Tail	Boundary	Within Phrase	Within Clause	Boundary
G1			G1			G1	ONcN – NcAdj N Pr	SVO'	
J1		J1					C - Pron	C – SAVO	
J3			J3				D – Adj N Pr Pron	c SAVO	
M2		M2					D – NPr V (sub. cl.)	c SVO'	
Q2		Q2					DNPr – Adj Nc Adj N	SVO	
Q3		Q3					DNPr – Adj Nc Adj N	SVO	
Q5		Q5					DNPr Adj NcAdj N	SVO	
R1						R1	DNPr Adj Nc – Adj N	SVO	
S2		S2					DNPr Adj Nc Adj N	SVO	
V1						V1			–A'SVO

Fig. 11. Chart: Profile of stuttering behaviour, Section 3 Pauses

References

Abbreviations

BJDC	*British Journal of Disorders of Communication*
B.J. Psychiat.	*British Journal of Psychiatry*
J.CH.Lang.	*Journal of Child Language*
JSHD	*Journal of Speech and Hearing Disorders*
JSHR	*Journal of Speech and Hearing Research*
JFD	*Journal of Fluency Disorders*

ABERCROMBIE, D. 1965: *Studies in phonetics and linguistics*. London: Oxford University Press.

— 1968: Some functions of silent stress. *Work in progress* **2**, Department of Phonetics and Linguistics, Edinburgh University, 1–11.

ADAMS, M.R. 1974: A physiologic and aerodynamic interpretation of fluent and stuttered speech. *JFD* **1**, 35–47.

ADAMS, M.R., FREEMAN, F.J. and CONTURE, E.G. (1985): Laryngeal dynamics of stutterers. In Curlee, R.F. and Perkins, W.H. (eds) *Nature and Treatment of Stuttering: New Directions*. London: Taylor and Francis, 89–129.

ADAMS, M.R. and HUTCHINSON, J. 1974: The effects of three levels of auditory masking on selected vocal characteristics and the frequency of disfluency of adult stutterers. *JSHR* **17**, 682–8.

ADAMS, M.R. and MOORE, W.H. 1972: The effects of auditory masking on the anxiety level, frequency of disfluency and selected vocal characteristics of stutterers. *JSHR* **15**, 572–8.

ADAMS, M.R. and REIS, R. 1971: The influence of the onset of phonation on the frequency of stuttering. *JSHR* **14**, 639–44.

— 1975: A reply to Martin Young. *JSHR* **18** 602–5.

ADAMS, M.R. and RUNYAN, C.M. 1981; Stuttering and fluency: exclusive events or points on a continuum. *JFD* **6**, 197–218.

AINSWORTH, C. 1939: Studies in the psychology of stuttering, 12: empathic breathing of auditors while listening to stuttering speech. *Journal of Speech Disorders* **4**, 149–56.

ALLEN, G.D. 1972: The location of rhythmic stress beats in English speech. Parts 1 and 2. *Language and Speech* **15**, 72–100, 179–95.

— 1975: Speech rhythm: its relation to performance universals and articulatory timing. *J. Phonetics* **3**, 75–86.

AMERMAN, J.D., DANILOFF, R. and MOLL, K. 1970: Lip and jaw coarticulation for the phoneme /æ/. *JSHR* **13**, 147–61.

AMMONS, R. and JOHNSON, W. 1944: Studies in the psychology of stuttering: 18, the construction and application of a test of attitudes towards stuttering. *J. Speech Disorders* **9**, 39–49.

ANDREWS, G., CRAIG, A., FEYER, A-M, HODDINOTT, S., HOWIE, P., and NEILSON, M. 1983: A review of research findings and theories circa 1982. *JSHD* **48**, 226–246.

ANDREWS, G. and CUTLER, J. 1974: Stuttering therapy: the relationship between changes in symptom level and attitudes. *JSHD* **39**, 312–19.

ANDREWS, G. and HARRIS, M. 1964: *The Syndrome of Stuttering*. London: Spastics Society Medical Education and Information Unit.

ANDREWS, G. and INGHAM, R. 1971: Stuttering: considerations in the evaluation of treatment. *BJDC* **6**, 129–38.

— 1972: An approach to the evaluation of stuttering therapy. *JSHR* **15**, 296–302.

ARGYLE, M. 1975: *Bodily Communication*. London: Methuen.

ARNOLD, G.E. 1960: Studies in tachyphemia: I, present concepts of etiologic factors. *Logos* **3c**, 25–45.

BARBARA, D.A. (ed.) 1962: *The Psychotherapy of Stuttering*. Springfield, Ill: Charles C. Thomas.

— (ed.) 1965: *New Directions in Stuttering: Theory and Practice*. Springfield, Ili: Charles C. Thomas.

BARIK, H.C. 1968: On defining juncture pauses: a note on Boomer's 'Hesitation and grammatical encoding'. *Language and Speech* **11**, 156–9.

BEECH, H.R. and FRANSELLA, F. 1968: *Research and Experiment in Stuttering*. London: Pergamon.

BERLIN, S. and BERLIN, C. 1964: Acceptability of stuttering control patterns. *JSHD* **29**, 436–41.

BERNSTEIN, N. 1967: *The Co-ordination and Regulation of Movements*. London: Pergamon.

BEVERIDGE, W.I.B. 1961: *The Art of Scientific Investigation*. London: Mercury Books.

BLOODSTEIN, O.N. 1960a: Development of stuttering, 1. *JSHD* **25**, 219–37.

— 1960b: Development of stuttering, 2. *JSHD* **25**, 366–76.

— 1961: Development of stuttering, 3. *JSHD* **26**, 67–82.

BLOODSTEIN, O.N. 1970: Stuttering and normal non-fluency—a continuity hypothesis. *BJDC* **5**, 30–9.

— 1974: The rules of early stuttering. *JSHD* **34**, 379–94.

BLOODSTEIN, O. 1981: *A Handbook on Stuttering*. 3rd ed. Chicago: National Easter Seal Society.

BLOODSTEIN, O.N., ALPER, J. and ZISK, P. 1965: Stuttering as an outgrowth of normal disfluency. In Barbara 1965, 31–54.

BLUEMEL, C.S. 1932: Primary and secondary stammering. *Quarterly J. Speech* **18**, 187–200.

BOBERG, E. (ed.) 1981: *Maintenance of Fluency*. New York, Oxford: Elsevier.

BOEHMLER, R.M., 1958: Listener responses to non-fluencies. *JSHR* **1**, 132–41.

BOHR, J.W.F. 1963: The effects of electronic and other external control methods on stuttering: a review of some research techniques and suggestions for further research. *J. South African Logopedic Society* **10**, 4–13.

BOOMER, D.S. 1965: Hesitation and grammatical encoding. *Language and Speech* **8**, 148–58.

— 1970: Review of F. Goldman-Eisler, *Psycholinguistic Experiments in Spontaneous Speech*. *Lingua* **25**, 152–64.

BOOMER, D.S. and DITTMAN, A.T. 1962: Hesitation pauses and juncture pauses in speech. *Language and Speech* **5**, 215–20.

BOOMER, D.S. and LAVER, J.D.M. 1968: Slips of the tongue. *BJDC* **3**, 2–12.

BOTTERILL, W. and COOK, F. 1987: Personal construct theory and the treatment of adolescent disfluency. In: L. Rustin, H. Purser, D. Rowley (eds.), *Progress in the Treatment of Fluency Disorders*. London, New York, Philadelphia: Taylor & Francis.

BOWMAN, J.P. 1971: *The Muscle Spindle and Neural Control of the Tongue*. Springfield, Ill: Charles C. Thomas.

BRAIN, R. 1960: *Clinical Neurology*. London: Oxford University Press.

BRANDON, S. and HARRIS, M. 1967: Stammering: an experimental treatment programme using syllable-timed speech. *BJDC* **2**, 64–8.

BRAZIER, M.A.B. 1960: Long-persisting electrical traces in the brain of man and their possible relationship to higher nervous activity. In H.H. Jasper and G.D. Smirnov (eds.), *The Moscow Colloquium on Electroencephalography of Higher Nervous Activity. Electroencephalography Journal Suppl.* **13**, 347–58.

BROOK, F. 1957: *Stammering and its Treatment.* London: Pitman.

BROWN, R. 1973: *A first language.* London: Allen and Unwin.

BROWN, R. and MCNEILL, D. 1966: The 'tip of the tongue' phenomenon. *J. Verbal Learning and Verbal Behaviour* **5**, 325–37.

BROWN, S.F. 1937: The influence of grammatical function on the incidence of stuttering. *J Speech Dis.* **2**, 207–215.

BROWN, S.F. 1938: Stuttering with relation to word accent and word position. *J. Abnormal Social Psychology* **33**, 112–20.

— 1945: The loci of stuttering in the speech sequence. *JSHD* **10**, 181–92.

— 1969: The loci of stuttering in the speech sequence. In O. Bloodstein (ed.), *A Handbook on Stuttering.* Chicago: National Easter Seal Society for Crippled Children and Adults.

BRUTTEN, G. 1982: Speech situation checklist for children: a discriminant analysis. Paper presented to the annual meeting of the *American Speech Language Hearing Association.* Toronto, Ontario.

BUTCHER, A. 1973: Pausen. *Arbeitsberichte* **1**, Institut für Phonetik, University of Kiel, 19–39.

— 1975: Some syntactic and physiological aspects of pausing. *Arbeitsberichte* **5**, Institut für Phonetik, Universiy of Kiel, 170–94.

CALDER, M. 1970: *The Mind of Man.* London: BBC.

CHEASMAN, C. 1983: Therapy for adults: an evaluation of current techniques for establishing fluency. In: P. Dalton (ed.), *Approaches to the Treatment of Stuttering.* London and Canberra: Croom Helm.

CHERRY, C. and SAYERS, B. 1956: Experiments upon the total inhibition of stammering by external control, and some clinical results. *J. Psychosomatic Research* **1**, 233–46.

CHOMSKY, C. 1969: *The Acquisition of Syntax in Children from 5 to 10.* Cambridge, Mass: MIT Press.

CHOMSKY, N. 1965: *Aspects of the Theory of Syntax.* Cambridge, Mass: MIT Press.

CHRISTENSEN, A. 1974: *Luria's Neuropsychological Investigation* (1st. Edition). Vojens: Schmilts Bogtrykkeri.

CLARK, R.M. and FITZPATRICK, J.A. 1962: Self-concepts in diagnosis and therapy. In Barbara 1962, 160–88.

CLARK, R.M. and MURRAY, F.P. 1965: Alterations in self-concept: a barometer of progress in individuals undergoing therapy for stuttering. In Barbara 1965, 131–58.

COLLEGE OF SPEECH THERAPISTS 1959: *Terminology for Speech Disorders.* London.

CONTURE, E.G. 1982: *Stuttering.* Englewood Cliffs, New Jersey: Prentice-Hall.

CONTURE, E.G. and BRAYTON, E.R. 1975: The influence of noise on stutterers' different disfluency types. *JSHR* **18**, 381–4.

CONTURE, E.G. and CARUSO, A.J. 1987: Assessment and diagnosis of childhood disfluency. In: L. Rustin, H. Purser, D. Rowley (eds.), *Progress in the Treatment of Fluency Disorders.* London, New York, Philadelphia: Taylor & Francis.

COOPER, E.B. 1979: Intervention procedures for the young stutterer. In: H.H. Gregory (ed.), *Controversies about Stuttering Therapy.* Baltimore: University Park Press.

COOPER, E.B. 1972: Recovery from stuttering in a junior and senior high school population. *JSHR* **15**, 632–8.

COOPER, S. 1960: Muscle spindles and other muscle receptors. In Bourne, G.H. (ed.), *Structure and Function of Muscle* **1**. New York: Academic Press, 381–420.

CORIAT, E.H. 1927: The oral-erotic components of stammering. *Int. J. Psychoanalysis* **8**, 56–69.

— 1931: The nature and analytical treatment of stuttering. *Proc. American Speech Correction Association* **1**, 151–6.

— 1943: The psychoanalytic concept of stammering. *Nervous Child* **2**, 167–71.

COSTELLO, J.M. and INGHAM, R.J. 1985: Assessment strategies for stuttering. In Curlee, R.F. and Perkins, W.H. (eds.) *Nature and Treatment of Stuttering: New Directions.* London: Taylor and Francis, 303–333.

CRUTTENDEN, A. 1974: An experiment involving comprehension of intonation in children from 7 to 10. *J.Ch.Lang.* **1**, 221–31.

CRYSTAL, D. 1969: *Prosodic System and Intonation in English.* Cambridge: Cambridge University Press.

— 1971: Stylistics, fluency and language teaching. In *Interdisciplinary approaches to language.* London: Centre for Information on Language Teaching, occasional paper **6**, 34–53.

— 1975: *The English Tone of Voice: Essays in Intonation, Prosody and Paralanguage.* London: Edward Arnold.

— 1976: *Child Language, Learning and Linguistics.* London: Edward Arnold.

— 1982: *Profiling Linguistic Disability.* London: Edward Arnold.

CRYSTAL, D. and DAVY, D. 1969: *Investigating English Style.* London: Longman.

CRYSTAL, D., FLETCHER, P. and GARMAN, M. 1976: *The Grammatical Analysis of Language Disability: a Procedure for Assessment and Remediation.* London: Edward Arnold.

CURLEE, R. 1984: Stuttering disorders: An overview. In Costello, J.M. (ed.) *Speech Disorders in Children: Recent Advances.* San Diego: College Hill Press.

DALTON, P. 1983: *Approaches to the Treatment of Stuttering.* London and Canberra. Croom Helm.

— 1986: A personal construct approach to therapy with children. In: G. Edwards (ed.), *Current Issues in Clinical Psychology.* New York, London: Plenum Press.

— 1988: The mother the child and the therapist: growing together. Paper presented at the *BPS Conference,* Leeds.

DANILOFF, R.G. and HAMMARBERG, R.E. 1973: On defining coarticulation. *J. Phonetics* **1**, 239–48.

DARLEY, F.L., ARONSON, A.E. and BROWN, J.R. 1969a: Differential diagnostic patterns of dysarthria. *JSHR* **12**, 246–69.

— 1969b: Clusters of deviant speech dimensions in the dysarthrias. *JSHR* **12**, 462–96.

— 1975: *Motor Speech Disorders.* Philadelphia and London: W.B. Saunders.

DORMAN, M.F. and PORTER, R.J. 1975: Hemispheric lateralization for speech perception in stutterers. *Cortex* **11**, 181–5.

DRAPER, M. 1968: Aids to improving vocalization. *New Zealand J. Physiotherapy* **3**, 11–17.

DREVER, J. 1952: *A Dictionary of Psychology.* London: Penguin.

DUFFY, R.J., HUNT, M.F. and GIOLAS, T.G. 1975: Effects of four types of disfluency on listener reactions. *Folia Phoniatrica* **27**, 106–15.

ECCLES, J.C. 1973: *The Understanding of the Brain.* New York: McGraw-Hill.

EDWARDS, M.L. 1974: Perception and production in child phonology: the testing of four hypotheses. *J.Ch.Lang.* **1**, 205–19.

EDWARDS, S. and HARDCASTLE, W. 1987: Linguistic profiling of stuttering behaviour. In Rustin, L., Purser, H. and Rowley, D. (eds.) *Progress in the Treatment of Fluency Disorders.* London: Taylor and Francis. 61–83.

EISENSON, J. (ed.) 1958: *Stuttering: a Symposium.* New York and Evanston: Harper and Row.

ERIKSON, R.L. 1969: Assessing communication attitudes among stutterers. *JSHR* **12**, 711–24.

FAIRBANKS, G. 1954: A theory of the speech mechanism as a servosystem. *JSHD* **19**, 133–9.

FAWCUS, M. 1970: Intensive treatment and group therapy for the child and adult stammerer. *BJDC* **5**, 59–65.

FENICHEL, O. 1945: *The Psychoanalytic Theory of Neurosis.* New York: Norton.

FLORANCE, C.L. and SHAMES, G.H. 1980: Stuttering treatment: issues in transfer and maintenance. *Seminars in Speech, Language and Hearing.* **1**, 375–388.

FOURCIN, A. and ABBERTON, E. 1971: First applications of a new laryngograph. *Medical and Biological Illustration* **21**, 172–82.

FRANSELLA, F. 1968: Self-concepts and the stutterer. *B.J. Psychiat.* **114**, 1531–5.

— 1970: Stuttering: not a symptom but a way of life. *BJDC* **5**, 22–9.

— 1972: *Personal Change and Reconstruction*. London and New York: Academic Press.

FREEMAN, F.J., USHIJIMA, T., DORMAN, M.F. and BORDEN, G.J. 1975: Disfluency and phonation: an electromyographic investigation of laryngeal activity accompanying the moment of stuttering. *Preprints of the 8th International Congress of Phonetic Sciences* (Leeds 1975).

FREUND, H. 1952: Studies in the interrelationship between stuttering and cluttering. *Folia Phoniatrica* **4**, 146–68.

FRIES, C.C. 1952: *The Structure of English*. New York: Harcourt Brace Jovanovich.

FROESCHELS, E. 1946: Cluttering. *J. Speech Disorders* **11**, 31–3.

FROMKIN, V.A. 1968: Speculations on performance models. *J. Linguistics* **4**, 47–68.

— 1971: The non-anomalous nature of anomalous utterances. *Language* **47**, 27–52.

— (ed.) 1973: *Speech Errors as Linguistic Evidence*. (Janua Linguarum, Series Maior 77.) The Hague: Mouton.

FRY, D.B. 1966: The development of the phonological system in the normal and deaf child. In F. Smith and G. Miller (eds.), *The Genesis of Language*. Cambridge, Mass: MIT Press, 187–206.

GAMMON, S.A., SMITH, P., DANILOFF, R. and KIM, C. 1971: Articulation and stress/juncture production under oral anæsthetization and masking. *JSHR* **14**, 271–82.

GESELL, A. 1954: *The First Five Years of Life*. London: Methuen.

GIMSON, A.C. 1970: *An Introduction to the Pronunciation of English*, 2nd edn. London: Edward Arnold.

GASNER, P.J. and VERMILYEA, F.D. 1953: An investigation of the definition and use of the diagnosis, 'primary stuttering'. *JSHD* **18**, 161–7.

GLAUBER, I.P. 1958: The psychoanalysis of stuttering. In Eisenson, 71–119.

GOLDIAMOND, I. 1965: Stuttering and fluency as manipulatable operant response classes. In L. Krasnar and L.P. Ullman (eds.), *Research and Behaviour Modification*. New York: Holt, Rinehart and Winston, 106–56.

GOLDMAN-EISLER, F. 1958: Speech production and the predictability of words in context. *Quarterly J. Experimental Psychology* **10**, 96–106.

— 1961a: Hesitation and information in speech. in C. Cherry (ed.), *Information Theory*. London: Butterworth, 162–74.

— 1961b: A comparative study of two hesitation phenomena. *Language and Speech* **4**, 18–26.

— 1968: *Psycholinguistics: Experiments in Spontaneous Speech*. London and New York: Academic Press.

— 1972: Pauses, clauses, sentences. *Language and Speech* **15**, 103–13.

GOLDSTEIN, K. 1948: *Language and Language Disorders*. New York: Grune and Stratton.

GOODGLASS, H. 1973: Studies on the grammar of aphasics. In H. Goodglass and S. Blumstein (eds.), *Psycholinguistics and Aphasia*. Baltimore: John Hopkins University Press, 183–218.

GREENE, M.C.L. 1964: *The Voice and its Disorders*. London: Pitman.

GREGORY, H.H. (ed.) 1979: *Controversies about Stuttering Therapy*. Baltimore: University Park Press.

GREGORY, H.H. 1986: Stuttering: a contemporary perspective. *Folia Phoniat.* **38**, 89–120.

GREGORY, H. and HILL, D. 1984: Stuttering therapy for children. In Perkins, W. *Stuttering Disorders*. New York: Thieme-Stratton.

GUITAR, B. 1974: Treatment of stuttering: electromyographic feedback for reduction of pre-utterance muscle action potentials. Conference Paper, American Speech and Hearing Association (Las Vegas, Nevada).

— 1975: Reduction of stuttering frequency, using analog electromyographic feed-back. *JSHR* **18**, 672–85.

GUITAR, B. and PETERS, T.J. 1980: *Stuttering: an Integration of Contemporary Theories*.

Memphis: Speech Foundation of America.

HADFIELD, J.A. 1962: *Childhood and Adolescence*. London: Pelican.

HALLIDAY, C.E. 1985: Stuttering as a cognitive-linguistic disorder. In Curlee, R.F. and Perkins, W.H. (eds.) *Nature and Treatment of Stuttering: New Directions*. London: Taylor and Francis. 259.

HAMRE C.E. 1985: Stuttering as a cognitive-linguistic disorder. In Curlee, R.F. and Perkins, W.H. (eds) *Nature and Treatment of Stuttering: New Directions* London: Taylor and Francis. 237-257.

HANNAH, E.P. and GARDNER, J.G. 1968: A note on syntactic relationships in nonfluency. *JSHD* **11**, 853-860.

HARDCASTLE, W.J. 1972: The use of electropalatography in phonetic research. *Phonetica* **25**, 197-215.

— 1974: Instrumental investigations of lingual activity during speech: a survey. *Phonetica* **29**, 129-57.

— 1975: Some aspects of speech production under controlled conditions of oral anaesthesia and auditory masking. *J. Phonetics* **3**, 197-214.

— 1976: *Physiology of Speech Production: an Introduction for Speech Scientists*. London: Academic Press.

HARDY, J.C. 1967: Suggestions for physiological research in dysarthria. *Cortex* **3**, 128-56.

HARRIS, K.S. 1974; Physiological aspects of articulation behaviour. In Sebeok, T. (ed.), *Current trends in linguistics* **12**. The Hague: Mouton, 2281-302.

HARRIS, K.S., LYSAUGHT, G.F. and SCHVEY, M.M. 1965: Some aspects of the production of oral and nasal labial stops. *Language and Speech* **8**, 135-47.

HAWKINS, P.R. 1971: The syntactic location of hesitation pauses. *Language and Speech* **14**, 277-88.

HAYHOW, R. 1983: The assessment of stuttering and the evaluation of treatment. In P. Dalton (ed.) *Approaches to the Treatment of Stuttering*. London and Canberra: Croom Helm.

HAYHOW, R. and LEVY, C. 1989: *Working with Stuttering: a Personal Construct Theory Approach*. Bicester: Winslow Press.

HEBB, D.O. 1949: *The Organization of Behaviour*. New York: Wiley.

HEILPERN, E. 1941: A case of stuttering. *Psychoanalytic Quarterly* **1**, 95-115.

HELMREICH, H.G. and BLOODSTEIN, O. 1973: The grammatical factor in childhood disfluency in relation to the continuity hypothesis. *JSHR* **16**, 731-8.

HENDERSON, A., GOLDMAN-EISLER, F. and SKARBECK, A. 1965: Temporal patterns of cognitive activity and breath control in speech. *Language and Speech* **8**, 236-42.

— 1966: Sequential temporal patterns in spontaneous speech. *Language and Speech* **9**, 207-16.

HIRSCH, K. de 1961: Studies in tachyphemia; 4, diagnosis of developmental language disorders. *Logos* **4**, 3-9.

HIXON, T.J. 1966: Turbulent noise sources for speech. *Folia Phoniatrica* **18**, 168-82.

HORII, Y., HOUSE, A.S., LI, K-P and RINGEL, R.L. 1973: Acoustic characteristics of speech produced without oral sensation. *JSHR* **16**, 67-77.

HUDGINS, C.V. and STETSON, R.H. 1937: Relative speed of articulatory movements. *Archives Néerlandaises de phonétique Expérimentale* **13**, 85-94.

HUSÉN, T. 1969: International impact of evaluation. In R.W. Tyler (ed.), *Educational Evaluation: New Roles, New Means*. University of Chicago Press, 335-50.

INGHAM, R.J. 1975: A comparison of covert and overt assessment procedures in stuttering therapy: outcome evaluation. *JSHR* **18**, 346-54.

— 1979: Comment on "Stuttering Therapy": the relation between attitude change and long-term outcome. *JSHD* **44**, 397-400.

— 1984: *Stuttering and Behaviour Therapy: Current Status and Experimental Foundations*. San Diego: College Hill Press.

INGRAM, D. 1976: *Phonological Disability in Children*. London: Edward Arnold.

INSKO, C.A. 1967: *Theories of Attitude Change*. New York: Appleton-Century-Crofts.

IRWIN, A. 1972: The treatment and results of 'easy stammering'. *BJDC* 7, 151–6.

JACKSON, J.H. 1932: On the nature of duality of the brain. In J. Taylor (ed.), *Selected Writings of John Hughlings Jackson*. London: Hodder and Stoughton.

JACKSON, S. and BANNISTER, D. 1985: Growing into self. In: D. Bannister (ed.), *Issues and Approaches in Personal Construct Theory*. London, Orlando, San Diego, New York, Toronto, Montreal, Sydney, Tokyo: Academic Press.

JAKOBSON, R. and HALLE, M. 1956: *Fundamentals of Language*. The Hague: Mouton.

JOHNSON, N.F. 1965: The psychological reality of phrase-structure rules. *J. Verbal Learning and Verbal Behaviour* 4, 469–75.

JOHNSON, W. 1939: The treatment of stuttering. *J. Speech Disorders* 4, 170–2.

— 1959: *The Onset of Stuttering: Research Findings and Implications*. Minneapolis: University of Minnesota Press.

— 1961: Measurements of oral reading and speaking rate and disfluency of college-age male and female stutterers and non-stutterers. *JSHD*, monograph suppl. 7, 1–20.

JOHNSON, W. and BROWN, S.F. 1935: Stuttering in relation to various speech sounds. *Quarterly Journal of Speech*, 21, 481–96.

JOHNSON, W., DARLEY, F.L. and SPRIESTERBACH, D.C. 1963: *Diagnostic Methods in Speech Pathology*. New York, Evanston and London: Harper and Row.

JOHNSON, W., NEELLEY, J.N., SANDER, E.K., WINITZ, H. and YOUNG, M.A. 1961: Studies of speech disfluency and rate of stutterers and non-stutterers. *JSHD*, monograph suppl. 7.

KAIDA, J. 1930: Über das Wesen das Stotterns (On the nature of stuttering). *Folia Oto-Laryngologica* 20.

KAPLAN, H.M. 1971: *Anatomy and Physiology of Speech*, 2nd ed. New York: McGraw-Hill.

KELHAM, R. 1978: An account of the experimental use of language teaching equipment in the treatment of children. (unpublished)

KELLY, G.A. 1955: *The Psychology of Personal Constructs*, 1 and 2. New York: Norton.

KIM, C.-W. 1971: Experimental phonetics: restropect and prospect. In W.O. Dingwell (ed.), *A Survey of Linguistic Science*. University of Maryland Press, 16–128.

KOZHEVNIKOV, V.A. and CHISTOVICH, L.A. 1965: *Rech: Artikulyatsiya i Vospriyatiye* (Speech: articulation and perception). Moscow and Leningrad: Nauka. (Translation by Joint Publications Research Service, US Dept of Commerce, Washington, DC, 30, 543.)

KRAUSE, M.S. and PILISUK, M. 1961: Anxiety in verbal behaviour: a validation study. *J. Consulting Psychology* 25, 414–19.

KUGELBERG, E. 1952: Facial reflexes. *Brain* 75, 385–96.

LADEFOGED, P. 1967: *Three Areas of Experimental Phonetics*. London: OUP.

— 1975: *A Course in Phonetics*. New York: Harcourt Brace Jovanovich.

LALLJEE, M.G. and COOK, M. 1969: An experimental investigation of the function of filled pauses in speech. *Language and Speech* 12, 24–8.

LANGOVÁ, J. and MORÁVEK, M. 1964: Some results of experimental examinations among stutterers and clutterers. *Folia Phoniatrica* 16, 290–6.

LASHLEY, K.S. 1951: The problem of serial order in behaviour. In L.A. Jeffress (ed.), *Cerebral Mechanisms in Behaviour*. New York: Wiley. (Reprinted in S. Saporta (ed.) 1961: *Psycholinguistics: a book of readings*. New York: Holt Rinehart and Winston, 180–98.)

LASZEWSKI, Z. 1956: Role of the department of rehabilitation in preoperative evaluation of Parkinsonian patients. *J. American Geriatric Society* 4, 1280–4.

LAVER, J.D.M.H. 1968: Phonetics and the brain. *Work in progress* 2, Department of Phonetics and Linguistics, University of Edinburgh, 63–75.

— 1969: The detection and correction of slips of the tongue. *Work in progress* 3, Department of Phonetics and Linguistics, University of Edinburgh, 1–12.

— 1970: The production of speech. In J. Lyons (ed.), *New Horizons in Linguistics*. London: Penguin, 53–75.

— 1977: Neurolinguistic aspects of speech production. In C. Gutknecht (ed.), *Grundbegriffe und Hauptströming der Linguistik*. Hamburg: Hoffmann und Campe.

LAY, C.H. and PAIVIO, A. 1969: The effects of task difficulty and anxiety on hesitations in speech. *Canadian J. Behavioural Science* **1**, 25–37.

LEBRUN, Y. and BOERS-VAN DIJK, M.B. 1973: Stuttering: a post-conference review. In Y. Lebrun and R. Hoops (eds.), *Neurolinguistic approaches to stuttering*. The Hague: Mouton, 133–7.

LEE, B.S. 1951: Artificial stutter. *JSHD* **16**, 53–65.

LEESON, R. 1975: Fluency and language teaching. London: Longman.

LENNEBERG, E.H. 1967: *Biological Foundations of Language*. London: Wiley.

LEVIN, H., SILVERMAN, I. and FORD, B.L. 1967: Hesitations in children's speech during explanation and description. *J. Verbal Learning and Verbal Behaviour* **6**, 560–4.

LEVY, C. (ed.) 1987: *Stuttering Therapies: Practical Approaches*. London, New York, Sydney: Croom Helm.

LIBERMAN, A.M., COOPER, F.S., HARRIS, K.S., MACNEILAGE, P.F. and STUDDERT-KENNEDY, M.G. 1967: Some observations on a model for speech perception. In W. Wathern-Dunn (ed.), *Models for the Perception of Speech and Visual Form*. Cambridge, Mass: MIT Press, 68–87.

LIEBMANN, A. 1900: *Vorlesungen Ueber Sprachstoerungen 4: Poltern (Paraphasia Praeceps)*. Berlin: Coblentz.

— 1930: Poltern, Paraphasia Praeceps. *Zeitschrift für die gesamte Neurologie und Psychiatrie* **127**.

LISKER, L. and ABRAMSON, A.S. 1964: A cross-language study of voicing in initial stops: acoustical measurements. *Word* **20**, 384–422.

LOUNSBURY, F.G. 1954: Transitional probability, linguistic structure and systems of habit-family hierarchies. In C.E. Osgood and T.A. Sebeok (eds.), *Psycholinguistics: A Survey of Theory and Research Problems*. Baltimore: Waverly, 93–101.

LOVE, L.R. and JEFFRESS, L.A. 1971: Identification of brief pauses in the fluent speech of stutterers and nonstutterers. *JSHR* **14**, 229–40.

LUCHSINGER, R. 1970: Inheritance of speech defects. *Folia Phoniartrica* **22**, 216–30.

LUCHSINGER, R. and LANDHOLT, H. 1951: Electroencephalographische Untersuchungen bei Stottern mit und ohne Polterkomponente. *Folia Phoniatrica* **3**, 135–51.

LURIA, A.R. 1970: *Traumatic Aphasia*. The Hague: Mouton.

MACKAY, D. and SODERBERG, G. 1970: The syllabic form of stuttered segments. Unpublished ms. University of California, Los Angeles.

MACLAY, H. and OSGOOD, C.E. 1959: Hesitation phenomena in spontaneous English speech. *Word* **15**, 19–44.

MACNEILAGE, P.F. 1970: Motor control of serial ordering of speech. *Psychological Review* **77**, 182–96.

— 1972: Speech psysiology. In J.H. Gilbert (ed.), *Speech and Cortical Functioning*. London: Academic Press, 1– 72.

MAHL, G.F. 1956: Disturbances and silences in patients' speech in psychotherapy. *J. Abnormal and Social Psychology* **53**, 1–15.

MARTIN, D.A. 1974: Some objections to the term 'apraxia of speech'. *JSHD* **39**, 53–64.

MARTIN, E., ROBERTS, K.H. and COLLINS, A.M. 1968: Short-term memory for sentences. *J. Verbal Learning and Verbal Behaviour* **7** 560–6.

MARRINER, N.A. and SANSON-FISHER, R.W. 1977: A behavioural approach to cluttering: a case study. *Australian J. Fl. Dis.* **5**, 134–141.

MARTIN, R.R., HAROLDSON, S.K. and TRIDEN, K.A. 1984: Stuttering and speech naturalness. *J.Speech and Hear Dis.* **49**, 53–58.

MATTHEWS, P.B.C. 1964: Muscle spindles and their motor control. *Physiological Review* **44**, 219–88.

— 1972: *Mammalian Muscle Receptors and Their Central Actions*. London: Edward Arnold.

MENYUK, P. 1971: *The Acquisition and Development of Language*. Englewood Cliffs, NJ: Prentice-Hall.

— 1972: *The Development of Speech*. Indianapolis: Bobbs-Merrill.

MERTON, P.A. 1953: Speculations on the servo-control of movement. In G.E.W. Wolstenholme (ed.), *The spinal cord*. London: Churchill, 247–55.

MILLER, G.A. and CHOMSKY, N. 1963: Finitary models of language users. In R. Luce, R. Bush and E. Galanter (eds.), *Handbook of Mathematical Psychology* **2**. New York: Wiley, 419–92.

MILLER, G.R. and HEWGILL, M.A. 1964: The effect of variations in non-fluency on audience ratings of source credibility. *Quarterly J. Speech* **50**. 36–44.

MILNER, P.M. 1970: *Physiological Psychology*. New York: Holt, Rinehart and Winston.

MINIFIE, F.D. and COOKER, H.S. 1964: A disfluency index. *JSHD* **10**, 189–92.

MITCHELL, T.F. 1969: Review of D. Abercrombie, *Elements of General Phonetics* (Edinburgh University Press). *J. Linguistics* **5**, 153–64.

MIYAKE, I. 1902: Researches on rhythmic action. In E.W. Scripture (ed.), *Studies from the Yale Psychological Laboratory* **10**. 1–48.

MOLL, K. and DANILOFF, R. 1971: Investigation of the timing of velar movements during speech. *J. Acoustical Society of America* **50**. 678–84.

MORLEY, M.E. 1957: *The Development and Disorders of Speech in Childhood*. Edinburgh: Livingstone.

MURRAY, D.C. 1971: Talk, silence and anxiety. *Psych. Bull.* **75**, 244–60.

NOOTEBOOM, S.G. 1969: The tongue slips into patterns. In A.G. Sciarone (ed.), *Nomen, Leyden studies in linguistics and phonetics*. The Hague: Mouton. 114–32.

O'CONNOR, J.D. and ARNOLD, G.F. 1973: *The Intonation of Colloquial English (2nd ed.)*. London: Edward Arnold.

ÖHMAN, S.E.G. 1966: Coarticulation in VCV utterances: spectrographic measurements. *J. Acoustical Society of America* **39**, 151–68.

PARKES, J.D. and MARSDEN, C.D. 1973: The treatment of Parkinson's disease. *British J. Hosptial Medicine* **10**. 284–94.

PEACHER, W.G. 1950: The etiology and differential diagnosis of dysarthria. *J. Speech Disorders* **15**, 252–65.

PERKINS, W.H. 1965: Stuttering: some common denominators. In Barbara 1965.

— 1981: Measurement and maintenance of Fluency. in: E. Boberg (ed.), *Maintenance of fluency*. New York, Oxford: Elsevier.

— 1983: The problem of definition: commentary on "stuttering". *JSHD* **48**, 246–249.

PIKE, K.L. 1945: *The Intonation of American English*. Ann Arbor: University of Michigan Press.

PRESTON, J.M. and GARDNER, R.C. 1967: Dimensions of oral and written language fluency. *J. Verbal Learning and Verbal Behaviour* **6**, 936–45.

QUINTING, G. 1971: *Hesitation Phenomena in Adult Aphasic and Normal Speech*. The Hague: Mouton.

QUIRK, R., GREENBAUM, S., LEECH, G. and SVARTVIK, J. 1972: *A Grammar of Contemporary English*. London: Longman.

QUIRK, R. and SVARTVIK, J. 1966: *Investigating Linguistic Acceptability*. The Hague: Mouton.

RAMER, A.L.H. 1976: Syntactic styles in emerging language. *J.Ch.Lang.* **3**, 49–62.

RAVENETTE, A.T. 1975: Grid techniques for children. *Journal of Child Psychlogy and Psychiatry*, **16**, 79–83.

— 1977: Personal construct theory: an approach to the psychological investigation of children and young people. In: D. Bannister (ed.) *New Perspectives in Personal Construct Theory*. London, New York, San Francsico: Academic Press.

— 1980: The exploration of consciousness: personal construct intervention with children.

In A. Lanfield and L. Leitner (eds.), *Personal Construct Psychology: Psychotherapy and Personality*. New York, Chichester, Brisbane, Toronto: Wiley.

REID, T. 1987: Intensive block modification therapy. In: C. Levy (ed.), *Stuttering Therapies: Practical Approaches*. London, New York, Sydney: Croom Helm.

REES, N. 1972: The role of babbling in the acquisition of language. *BJDC* **7**, 17–23.

REYNOLDS, A. and PAIVIO, A. 1968: Cognitive and emotional determinants of speech. *Canadian J. Psychology* **22**, 164–75.

RILEY, G. and RILEY, J. 1979: A component model for diagnosing and treating children who stutter. *J. Fl. D.* **4**, 279–293.

— 1982: Evaluating stuttering problems in children. In: H. Luper (ed.), *Intervention with the Young Stutterer. Journal of Childhood Communication Disorders*, **VI**, 15–25.

— 1983: Evaluation as a basis for intervention. In: D. Preins and R. Ingham (eds.), *Treatment of Stuttering in Early Childhood*. San Diego, CA: College-Hill

RINGEL, R.L. and STEER, M.D. 1963: Some effects of tactile and auditory alterations on speech output. *JSHR* **6**, 369–78.

ROBERTS, T.D.M. 1966: *Basic ideas in neurophysiology*. London: Butterworth.

ROBINSON, F.B. 1964: *Introduction to stuttering*. Englewood Cliffs, NJ: Prentice-Hall.

ROCHESTER, S.R. 1973: The significance of pauses in spontaneous speech. *J. Psycholinguistic Research* **2(1)**, 51–81.

RONSON, I. 1976: Word frequency and stuttering: the relationship to sentence structure. *JSHD* **19**, 813–819.

ROSENBEK, L., MCNEIL, M.R. and ARONSON, A.E. (eds.) 1984: *Apraxia of Speech*. San Diego: College-Hill.

ROSENBEK, J.C., LEMME, M.L., AHERN, M.B., HARRIS, E.H. and WERTZ, R.T. 1973: A treatment for apraxia of speech in adults. *JSHD* **38**, 462–72.

ROSENBERG, S. and CURTIS, J. 1954: The effect of stuttering on the behaviour of the listener. *J. Abnormal Psychology* **49**, 355–61.

RUDER, K.F. 1973: Duration of silent intervals as a perceptual cue of speech pauses. *Perceptual and Motor Skills* **36**, 47–57.

RUDER, K.F. and JENSEN, P.J. 1972: Fluent and hesitation pauses as a function of syntactic complexity. *JSHR* **15** 49–60.

RUSHWORTH, G. 1966: Some functional properties of deep facial afferents. In B.L. Andrew (ed.), *Control and Innervation of Skeletal Muscle*. Edinburgh: Livingstone, 125–33.

RUSTIN, L. and COOK, F. 1983: Intervention procedures for the disfluent child. In: P. Dalton (ed.), *Approaches to the Treatment of Stuttering*. London and Canberra: Croom Helm.

RUSTIN, L. and PURSER, H. 1984: Intensive treatment models for adolescent stuttering: social skills versus speech techniques. Proceedings of the *XIX Congress of the IALP*. Brussels: IALP.

RUSTIN, L., PURSER, H. and ROWLEY, D. (eds.) 1987: *Progress in the Treatment of Fluency Disorders*. London, New York, Philadelphia: Taylor & Francis.

RYAN, B.P. and VAN KIRK, B. 1974: The establishment, transfer and maintenance of fluent speech in 50 stutterers using delayed auditory feedback and operant procedures. *JSHD* **39**, 3–10.

SACHS, J. and DEVIN, J. 1976: Young children's use of age-appropriate speech styles in social interaction and role-playing. *J.Ch.Lang.* **3**, 81–98.

SALMON, P. 1976: Grid measures with child subjects. In: P. Slater (ed.) *Explorations of Intrapersonal Space*. London, New York, Sydney, Toronto: Wiley.

SANDER, E.K. 1961: Reliability of the Iowa speech disfluency test. *JSHD*, monograph suppl. **7**, 21–30.

— 1963: Frequency of syllable repetitions and 'stutter' judgements. *JSHD* **28**, 19–30.

SCHUELL, H., JENKINS, J.J. and JIMENEZ-PABON, E. 1964: *Aphasia in Adults: Diagnosis, Prognosis and Treatment*. New York, Evanston and London: Harper and Row, Hoeber

Medical Division.

SCOTT, C.M. and RINGEL, R.L. 1971; Articulation without oral sensory control. *JSHR* **14**, 804–18.

SEEMAN, M. 1951: Pathogenesis of stuttering. *La Presse médicale* **159**, 164–5.

SERENO, K.K. and HAWKINS, G.J. 1967: The effects of variations in speakers' non-fluency upon audience ratings of attitude toward the speech topic and speaker's credibility. *Speech Monograph* **34**, 121–66.

SHEEHAM, J.G. 1958: Conflict theory of stuttering. In: J. Eisenson (ed.), *Stuttering: a Symposium*. New York: Harper and Row, 121–66.

— (ed.) 1970: *Stuttering: Research and Therapy*. New York: Evanston and London: Harper and Row.

— 1974: Stuttering behaviour: a phonetic analysis. *J. Communication Disorders* **7**, 193–212.

— 1979: Current issues on stuttering and recovery. In: H.H. Gregory (ed.), *Controversies about Stuttering Therapy*. Baltimore: University Park Press.

SHEEHAN, J.G. and MARTYN, M.M. 1970: Stuttering and its disappearance. *JSHR* **13**, 279–89.

SHERIDAN, M.D. 1968: The developmental progress of infants and young children. *Reports on Public Health and Medical Subjects* **102**, London: HMSO.

SHINE, R.E. 1980: *Systematic Fluency Training for Young Children*. Tigard, OR: CC Publications.

SIGMAN, A.W. and POPE, B. 1965: Effects of question specificity and anxiety-producing messages on verbal fluency in the initial interview. *J. Personal Social Psychology* **2**, 522–30.

— 1966: Ambiguity and verbal fluency in the TAT. *J. Consulting Psychology* **30**, 239–45.

SILVERMAN, E. 1973: Generality of disfluency data collected from preschoolers. *JSHD* **16**, 474–481.

SILVERMAN, F.H. and GOODBAN, M.T. 1972: The effect of auditory masking on the fluency of normal speakers. *JSHR* **15**, 543–6.

SILVERMAN, F.H. and WILLIAMS, D.E. 1972: Prediction of stuttering by school-age stutterers. *JSHR* **15**, 189–93.

SMITH, A.H. and O'LOUGHLIN, J.L.N. (eds.): *Dictionary of the English language*. London: Odhams.

SMITH, N. 1974: The acquisition of phonological skills in children. *BJDC* **9**, 17–23.

SMITH, R.G. 1962: A semantic differential for speech correction concepts. *Speech Monographs* **29**, 32–7.

SMITH, T.S. and LEE, C.Y. 1972: Peripheral feedback mechanisms in speech production models. *Proc. 7th International Congress of Phonetic Sciences* 1199–1204. The Hague: Mouton.

SODERBERG, G.A. 1959: *A study of the effects of delayed auditory side-tone on four aspects of stutterers' speech during oral reading and spontaneous speaking*. PhD dissertation, Ohio State University.

— 1962: Phonetic influences upon stuttering. *JSHR* **5**, 315–19.

— 1966: The relations of stuttering to word length and word frequency. *JSHR* **9**, 584–9.

— 1967: Linguistic factors in stuttering. *JSHR* **10**, 801–810.

— 1968: Delayed auditory feedback and stuttering. *JSHD* **33**, 260–7.

— 1969: Delayed auditory feedback and the speech of stutterers: a review of studies. *JSHD* **34**, 20–9.

— 1971: Relation of word information and word length to stuttering disfluencies. *J.Comm.Dis* **4**, 9–14.

STARKWEATHER, C.W. ARMSON, J.M. and AMSTER, B.J. 1987: An approach to the study of motor speech mechanisms in stuttering. In Rustin, L., Purser, H. and Rowley, D. (eds.) *Progress in the Treatment of Fluency Disorders*. London: Taylor and Francis. 43–58.

STEIN, L. 1953: Stammering as a psychosomatic disorder. *Folia Phoniatrica* **5**, 12–46.

ST LOUIS, K.O. 1979: Linguistic and motor aspects of stuttering. In Lass, N.J. (ed.) *Speech and Language: Advances in Basic Research*, Vol. 1. New York: Academic Press.

ST LOUIS, K.O. and WESTBROOK, J.B. 1987: The effectiveness of treatment for stuttering. In: L. Rustin, H. Purser and D. Rowley (eds.) *Progress in the Treatment of Fluency Disorders*. London, New York, Philadelphia: Taylor & Francis.

SWEET, H. 1877: *A Handbook of Phonetics*. Oxford: Clarendon Press.

— 1890: *A Primer of Phonetics*. Oxford: Clarendon Press.

TATHAM, M.A.A. 1973: Implications on stuttering of a model of speech production. In: Y. Lebrun and R. Hoops (eds.), *Neurolinguistic Approaches to Stuttering*. The Hague: Mouton, 101–11.

TAYLOR, I. 1969: Content and structure in sentence production. *J. Verbal Learning and Verbal Behavior* **8**, 170–5.

THOMPSON, J. 1983: *Assessment of Fluency in School-Age Children*. Resource Guide. Danville, Il: Interstate Printers and Publishers.

TORNICK, G.B. and BLOODSTEIN, O. 1976: Stuttering and sentence length. *JSHR* **19** 651–654.

VALLBO, A.B. 1971: Muscle spindle response at the onset of isometric voluntary contractions in man: time difference between fusimotor and skelemotor effects. *Physiology* **218**, 405–31.

VAN DEN BERG, J. 1958: Myoelastic-aerodynamic theory of voice production. *JSHR* **1**, 227–44.

VAN RIPER, C. 1954: *Speech Correction*. Englewood Cliffs, NJ: Prentice-Hall.

— 1971: *The Nature of Stuttering*. (1st ed.) Englewood Cliffs, NJ: Prentice-Hall.

— 1973: *Treatment of stuttering*. Englewood Cliffs, NJ: Prentice-Hall.

— 1982: *The Nature of Stuttering*. (2nd ed.) Englewood Cliffs, NJ: Prentice-Hall.

WATTS, F. 1973: Mechanisms of fluency control in stutterers. *BJDC* **8**, 131–8.

WEBSTER, R.L. 1979: Empirical considerations regarding stuttering therapy. In: H.H. Gregory (ed.), *Controversies about Stuttering Therapy*. Baltimore: University Park Press.

WEINSTOCK, J.J. 1968: A child psychiatrist's view of therapy for stuttering. *JSHD* **33**, 15–20.

WEISS, D.A. 1960: The theory of cluttering. *Proc. 11th International Speech and Voice Therapy Conference*. Basel: Karger, 128–9.

— 1964: *Cluttering*. Englewood Cliffs, NJ: Prentice-Hall.

— 1967: Cluttering. *Folia Phoniatrica* **19**, 233–63.

WEPMAN, J. 1972: Aphasia therapy: a new look. *JSHD* **37**, 203–14.

WEST, R. 1958: An agnostic's speculations about stuttering. In Eisenson, 167–222.

WILKES, A.L. and KENNEDY, R.A. 1969: Relationship between pausing and retrieval latency in sentences of varying grammatical form. *J. Experimental Psychology* **79**, 241–5.

WILLIAMS, D., SILVERMAN, F.H. and KOOLS, J. 1968: Disfluency behaviour of elementary school stutterers: the adaptation effect. *JSHR* **11**, 622–30.

WILLIAMS, D.E. and KENT, L.R. 1958: Listener evaluations of speech interruptions. *JSHR* **1**, 124–31.

WILLIAMS, G.T., FARQUHARSON, I.M. and ANTHONY, J. 1975: Fibreoptic laryngoscopy in the assessment of laryngeal disorders. *J. Laryngology and Otology* **89**, 299–316.

WINGATE, M.E. 1964a: Recovery from stuttering. *JSHD* **29**, 312–21.

— 1964b: A standard definition of stuttering. *JSHD* **29** 484–489.

— 1967: Stuttering and word length. *JSHR* **10**, 146–52.

— 1969a: Sound and pattern in artificial fluency. *JSHR* **12**, 677–86.

— 1969b: Stuttering as phonetic transition defect. *JSHD* **34**, 107–8.

— 1970: Effect on stuttering of changes in audition. *JSHR* **13**, 861–73.

— 1985: Stuttering as a prosodic disorder. In Curlee, R.F. and Perkins, W.H. (eds.) *Nature and Treatment of Stuttering: New Directions*. London: Taylor and Francis. 215–235.

WISCHNER, G.J. 1950: Stuttering behaviour and learning. *JSHD* **15**, 324–34.

— 1952: Experimental approach to expectancy and anxiety in stuttering behaviour. *JSHD* **17**, 139–54.

— 1969: Stuttering behaviour, learning theory and behaviour therapy: problems, issues and progress. In B.B. Gray and G. England (eds.), *Stuttering and the Conditioning Therapies*. Monterey, Calif: Monterey Institute for Speech and Hearing.

WOHL, M.T. 1970: The treatment of non-fluent utterance—a behavioural approach. *BJDC* **5**, 66–76.

WOLK, L. 1986: Cluttering: a diagnostic case report. *BJDC*. **21**, 199–207.

WOLPE, J. 1969: Behaviour therapy of stuttering: deconditioning the emotional factor. in B.B. Gray and G. England (eds.), *Stuttering and the Conditioning Therapies*. Monterey, Calif: Monterey Institute for Speech and Hearing.

WOODROW, H. 1951; Time perception. In S.S. Stevens (ed.), *Handbook of Experimental Psychology*. New York: Wiley, 1224–36.

WOODS, C.L. 1974: Social position and speaking competence of stuttering and normally fluent boys. *JSHR* **17**, 740–7.

WOODS, C.L. and WILLIAMS. D.E. 1976: Traits attributed to stuttering and normally fluent males. *JSHR* **19**, 267–78.

WOOLF, G. 1967: The assessment of stuttering as struggle. avoidance and expectancy. *BJDC* **2**, 158–67.

YAIRI, E. and CLIFTON, N.F. Jr. 1972: Disfluent speech behaviour of preschool children, high school senior, and geriatric persons. *JSHR* **15**, 714–19.

YAIRI, E. and LEWIS, B. 1984: Disfluencies at the onset of stuttering. *JSHR* **27**, 154–159.

YORKSTON, K.M., BEUKELMAN, D.R. and BELL, K.R. 1987: *Clinical Management of Dysarthric Speech*. London: Taylor & Francis.

YOUNG, M.R. 1975a: Comment on stuttering frequency and the onset of phonation. *JSHR* **18**, 600–2.

— 1975b: Onset prevalence and recovery from stuttering. *JSHD* **40**, 49–58.

Index

Cole & Whurr Journals of related interest

THE BRITISH JOURNAL OF DISORDERS OF COMMUNICATION

The British Journal of Disorders of Communication is an academically
rigorous and intellectually challenging journal which presents the latest
clinical and theoretical research and is a principal forum for the discussion of
the entire range of communication disorders. The journal contains a
representative and balanced selection of articles, with contributions from
North America, Australasia and Continental Europe, as well as the UK.
Among the leading articles published in recent issues are:
August 1987: Duncan & Gibbs - Acquisition of Syntax in Panjabi and English
December 1987: Gibbon and Hardcastle - Articulatory Description and
Treatment of 'lateral /S/ using Electropalatography: A Case Study
April 1988: Perry - Surgical Voice Restoration following Laryngectomy: The
Tracheo-oesophageal fistula technique (Singer-Blom)
August 1988: Bryan - Assessment of Language Disorders after Right
Hemisphere Damage; Lebrun - Language and Epilepsy: A Review

The journal is owned by the College of Speech Therapists, and the Editor is
Elspeth McCartney of Glasgow University and Jordanhill College. Issues are
published three times a year and annual volumes are of up to 500 pages.

ISSN: 0007 098X

THE BRITISH JOURNAL OF EXPERIMENTAL AND CLINICAL HYPNOSIS

This is the Journal of the British Society of Experimental and Clinical
Hypnosis, a learned society which brings together appropriately qualified
medical professionals who have a legitimate reason for using hypnosis in their
work and who share a scientific interest in the research and practical
application of hypnosis. The journal provides a forum for the critical
discussion of ideas, theories, findings, procedures and social policies
associated with the topic of hypnosis. It also disseminates information on all
aspects of theory, research and practice. A book review section is included.

ISSN:0265 1033

Please send for the Cole & Whurr catalogue.

Cole & Whurr Ltd
19b Compton Terrace, London N1 2UN
01-359 5979

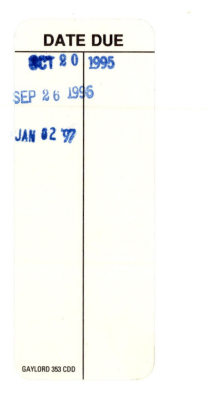